Hypotensive Syndromes in Geriatric Patients

Kannayiram Alagiakrishnan
Maciej Banach
Editors

Hypotensive Syndromes in Geriatric Patients

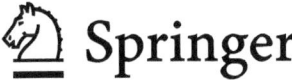 Springer

Editors
Kannayiram Alagiakrishnan
Division of Geriatric Medicine
University of Alberta
Edmonton, AB
Canada

Maciej Banach
Polish Mother's Memorial Hospital
Research Institute (PMMHRI)
Lodz, Poland

ISBN 978-3-030-30331-0   ISBN 978-3-030-30332-7   (eBook)
https://doi.org/10.1007/978-3-030-30332-7

This Springer imprint is published by the registered company Springer Nature Switzerland AG
The registered company address is: Gewerbestrasse 11, 6330 Cham, Switzerland

Disclaimer

The statements and opinions in this book are solely those of individual authors and contributors. The authors and editors have worked to ensure that all information in this book is consistent with accepted medical standards and practice at the time of publication. Medical standards can change and evolve because of new research and practice advancement. The reader is urged to check the package product insert for each drug for any change in indications and dosage as well as for added warnings and precautions. However, the authors, editors and publishers are not legally responsible for errors or omissions or any consequences from application of the information in this book.

Contents

Contributors

Ali Ahmed Washington DC VA Medical Center and George Washington University and Georgetown University, Washington, DC, USA

Kannayiram Alagiakrishnan Division of Geriatric Medicine, University of Alberta, Edmonton, AB, Canada

Wilbert S. Aronow, MD, FACC, FAHA Cardiology Division, Department of Medicine, Westchester Medical Center and New York Medical College, Valhalla, NY, USA

Maciej Banach Department of Hypertension, Chair of Nephrology and Hypertension, Medical University of Lodz, Lodz, Poland

Department of Cardiology and Congenital Diseases of Adults, Polish Mother's Memorial Hospital Research Institute (PMMHRI), Lodz, Poland

Marcin Adam Bartłomiejczyk Department of Hypertension, Medical University of Lodz, Lodz, Poland

Agata Bielecka-Dabrowa Department of Hypertension, Chair of Nephrology and Hypertension, Medical University of Lodz, Lodz, Poland

Department of Cardiology and Congenital Diseases of Adults, Polish Mother's Memorial Hospital Research Institute (PMMHRI), Lodz, Poland

Marlena Broncel Department of Internal Diseases and Clinical Pharmacology, Medical University of Lodz, Lodz, Poland

Adrian Covic Grigore T. Popa University of Medicine, Strada Universității, Iasi, Romania

Paulina Gorzelak-Pabiś Department of Internal Diseases and Clinical Pharmacology, Medical University of Lodz, Lodz, Poland

Anna Kasperowicz University Hospital, Clinical Department of Cardiology, Zielona Gora, Poland

Marek Maciejewski Department of Cardiology and Congenital Diseases of Adults, Polish Mother's Memorial Hospital Research Institute (PMMHRI), Lodz, Poland

Darren Mah University of Alberta, Edmonton, AB, Canada

Jolanta Malyszko Department of Nephrology, Dialysis and Internal Medicine, Warsaw Medical University, Warszawa, Poland

Kamal Masaki Division of Geriatric Medicine, University of Hawaii at Manoa, Honolulu, HI, USA

Mariusz Stasiolek, MD, PhD Department of Neurology, Medical University of Lodz, Lodz, Poland

Wilbert S. Aronow

Introduction

Orthostatic hypotension is diagnosed if there is a reduction of ≥ 20 mm in systolic blood pressure or of ≥ 10 mm in diastolic blood pressure within 3 minutes of standing [1–5]. Patients being treated with antihypertensive drugs should have their blood pressure measured in the sitting position and within 3 minutes of standing [2]. Their blood pressure should not be measured immediately after eating as postprandial hypotension may occur then [6, 7]. Orthostatic changes in blood pressure should be measured at 1 minute and at 3 minutes after standing [8, 9].

Disorders associated with orthostatic hypotension include advanced age and disorders associated with hypovolemia including anemia, overdiuresis, diarrhea, vomiting, poor food and fluid intake, hemorrhage, and reduced plasma volume [10]. Hypertension, diabetes mellitus, neurological disorders, cardiovascular disorders, endocrine disorders, alcoholism, vascular insufficiency, connective tissue disorders, vitamin B12 deficiency, uremia, amyloidosis, and porphyria are also associated with orthostatic hypotension. Drugs associated with orthostatic hypotension include alcohol, diuretics which may cause volume depletion, and vasodilators such as angiotensin-converting enzyme inhibitors, angiotensin receptor blockers, calcium channel blockers, hydralazine, nitrates, and prazosin which cause a decrease in systemic vascular resistance and venodilation. Centrally acting antihypertensive drugs such as alpha methyldopa, clonidine, guanethidine, hexamethonium, labetalol, mecamylamine, and phenoxybenzamine and drugs associated with torsades de pointes are associated with orthostatic hypotension. Antidepressants, antipsychotic drugs, anti-Parkinsonian medications are also associated with orthostatic hypotension [10]. One study showed that enalapril and nifedipine were equipotent in reducing blood pressure with enalapril reducing the number of orthostatic hypotensive

W. S. Aronow (✉)
Cardiology Division, Department of Medicine, Westchester Medical Center and New York Medical College, Valhalla, NY, USA

© Springer Nature Switzerland AG 2020
K. Alagiakrishnan, M. Banach (eds.), *Hypotensive Syndromes in Geriatric Patients*, https://doi.org/10.1007/978-3-030-30332-7_1

1

episodes and nifedipine increasing the number of orthostatic hypotensive episodes [11]. The functional adenine insertion polymorphism in the endothelin gene is not associated with hypertension or orthostatic hypotension in Chinese persons [12].

Pathophysiology

Orthostatic hypotension may be caused by an excessive decrease in blood volume when the person assumes an upright position or from inadequate cardiovascular compensation for a reduction in cardiac preload when the person assumes an upright position [13]. When changing from a lying to standing position, about 500 ml of blood pool in the lower extremities. Baroreceptors in the carotid sinus and aortic arch are sensitive to the reduction in arterial pressure with postural change, resulting in vagal inhibition and sympathetic stimulation [14]. Failure of these autonomic mechanisms may cause postural hypotension. Increased left ventricular stiffness with aging caused by increased interstitial fibrosis and cross linking of collagen in the heart impairs left ventricular diastolic relaxation and filling [15]. Conditions that further reduce left ventricular filling with a decrease in intravascular volume or decreased venous return to the heart when the person assumes the upright position, especially if they are receiving drugs which may contribute to orthostatic hypotension, may cause orthostatic hypotension [13–16].

Orthostatic hypotension in the elderly is associated with hypertension, impaired left ventricular filling, altered sympathovagal balance, increased left ventricular wall thickness, reduced left ventricular preload, and impaired diastolic filling of the left ventricle [16]. Hypertension predisposes to orthostatic hypotension by impairing baroreceptor reflex sensitivity and decreasing vascular and left ventricular compliance [13–16]. Alcohol potentiates orthostatic hypotension by impairing the vasoconstrictor response to orthostatic stress [17]. Impaired blood pressure stabilization is more common as we become older and was reported in the Irish Longitudinal Study on Ageing [18]. Middle-aged adults with orthostatic hypotension developed after 23-year follow-up echocardiographic left ventricular hypertrophy (hazard ratio = 1.97), reduced right chamber volume (hazard ratio = 1.74), and decreased early diastolic tissue velocity in the left ventricular septal wall (hazard ratio = 1.47), independent of traditional risk factors [19].

Prevalence

The prevalence of orthostatic hypotension in older persons was 8% in 476 persons [1]. In this study, the prevalence of orthostatic hypotension was 13% in 257 persons receiving cardiovascular or psychotropic drugs and 3% in 219 persons who did not receive cardiovascular or psychotropic drugs [1]. The prevalence of orthostatic hypotension was 15% in 168 patients [20], 18% of 5273 persons in the Cardiovascular Health Study [4], 17% of 100 persons [21], 22% in 186 persons [22], 17.8% at baseline, 10.4% at 1 year, 12.8% at 4 years, and 20.0% at 1 or more visits in 4733 diabetics in the Action to Control Cardiovascular Risk in Diabetes (ACCORD) blood pressure trial [23]. The prevalence of orthostatic hypotension in 4736 persons in the Systolic Hypertension in the Elderly Program cohort was 10.4% when measured at 1 minute after standing, 12.0% when measured at 3 minutes after standing, and 17.3% when measured at both 1 and 3 minutes after standing [8].

The prevalence of orthostatic hypotension in 9361 persons mean age 67.9 years, in the Systolic Blood Pressure Intervention Trial (SPRINT), was 16.6% in persons randomized to a systolic blood pressure below 120 mm Hg versus 18.3% in persons randomized to a systolic blood pressure below 140 mm Hg [24]. The prevalence of orthostatic hypotension in 2636 persons aged 75 years and older, mean age 79.9 years, in SPRINT was 21.0% in persons randomized to a systolic blood pressure below 120 mm Hg versus 21.8% in persons randomized to a systolic blood pressure below 140 mm Hg [25]. In this study, the prevalence of orthostatic hypotension with dizziness was 1.9% in persons randomized to a systolic blood pressure less than 120 mm Hg versus 1.3% in persons randomized to a systolic blood pressure less than 140 mm Hg [25].

Symptoms

Symptoms associated with orthostatic hypotension include dizziness, falls, fractures, light-headedness, and syncope [2, 3, 15, 26–36]. In a study of 4127 Irish persons, mean age 61.5 years, orthostatic hypotension was associated with an increased risk of unexplained falls (relative risk = 1.52), all-cause falls (relative risk = 1.40), and injurious falls (relative risk = 1.81) [34]. Of 352 patients, mean age 78 years, the etiology of syncope was diagnosed in 243 patients (69%) [35]. Of the 352 patients, vasovagal syncope was diagnosed in 12%, volume depletion in 14%, orthostatic hypotension in 5%, cardiac syncope in 29%, carotid sinus hypersensitivity in 2%, and drug overdose/others in 7% [35]. In a study of 11,429 participants followed for a median of 27 years, orthostatic hypotension was associated with dizziness (odds ratio = 1.49), falls (adjusted hazard ratio = 1.22), fractures (adjusted hazard ratio = 1.16), syncope (adjusted hazard ratio = 1.40), motor vehicle crashes (adjusted hazard ratio = 1.43), and all-cause mortality (adjusted hazard ratio = 1.36) [36].

Prognosis

The Honolulu Heart Program included 3522 elderly men [37]. The prevalence of orthostatic hypotension in this study was 6.9% and increased with age. At 4-year follow-up, orthostatic hypotension was significantly associated with increased all-cause mortality by 1.64 times [37]. The Cardiovascular Health Study included 5273 community-dwelling adults, mean age 73 years [4]. The prevalence of orthostatic hypotension was 18% in this study. We reported that propensity analysis of 883 persons with orthostatic hypotension and 2627 persons without orthostatic hypotension (mean age 74 years; 58% women) demonstrated at 13-year follow-up that orthostatic hypotension was significantly associated with incident heart failure by 1.24 times. Symptomatic orthostatic hypotension was significantly associated with incident heart failure by 1.57 times. Asymptomatic orthostatic hypotension was associated with incident heart failure by 1.17 times [4].

The Progetto Veneto Anziani (Pro.V.A.) study included 2786 community-dwelling Italians, mean age 76 years (59% women) [38]. The prevalence of orthostatic hypotension was 9.3% in this study. At 4.4-year follow-up, orthostatic hypotension was associated with increased all-cause mortality by 1.13 times [38]. The Swedish Malmo Preventive Project included 33, 346 persons, mean age 45.7 years (67% men) [39]. The prevalence of orthostatic hypotension was 6.2% in this study. At 22.7-year follow-up, orthostatic hypotension was significantly associated with all-cause mortality by 1.21 times, with coronary events by 1.17 times, with stroke by 1.17 times, and by the composite endpoint of death, coronary event, or stroke by 1.18 times [39].

The Orthostatic Hypotension in Diabetics in the Action to Control Cardiovascular Risk in Diabetes Blood Pressure (ACCORD BP) trial investigated the prevalence, incidence, and prognostic significance of orthostatic hypotension in the ACCORD BP trial [5, 23]. The 4266 participants, mean age 62.1 years (50% men), in this study were at high risk for orthostatic hypotension because they all had type 2 diabetes mellitus, hypertension, and were being treated with antihypertensive drugs. Orthostatic blood pressure measurements were made in 1321 persons at baseline, in 2625 persons at 12 months, in 3702 persons at 48 months, and in 926 persons at all 3 visits.

The prevalence of orthostatic hypotension was 17.8% at baseline, 10.4% at 12 months, 12.8% at 48 months, and 20% at one or more visits [23]. At baseline, the prevalence of orthostatic hypotension was 19.3% in hypertensive diabetics treated to a systolic blood pressure less than 120 mm Hg versus 16.1% in hypertensive diabetics treated to a systolic blood pressure less than 140 mm Hg (p not significant). At 12 months, the prevalence of orthostatic hypotension was 9.5% in hypertensive diabetics treated to a systolic blood pressure less than 120 mm Hg versus 11.4% in hypertensive diabetics treated to a systolic blood pressure less than 140 mm Hg (p not significant). At 48 months, the prevalence of orthostatic hypotension was 12.2% in hypertensive diabetics treated to a systolic blood pressure less than 120 mm Hg versus 13.5% in hypertensive diabetics treated to a systolic blood pressure less than 140 mm Hg (p not significant).

At 12 months, the incidence of orthostatic hypotension was 8.0% in hypertensive diabetics treated to a systolic blood pressure less than 120 mm Hg versus 9.9% in hypertensive diabetics treated to a systolic blood pressure less than 140 mm Hg (p not significant). At 48 months, the incidence of orthostatic hypotension was 9.9% in hypertensive diabetics treated to a systolic blood pressure less than 120 mm Hg versus 11.0% in hypertensive diabetics treated to a systolic blood pressure less than 140 mm Hg (p not significant). Dizziness upon standing for the blood pressure measurements was similar for both treatment groups at baseline and at 6 months but was higher with a systolic blood pressure less than 120 mm Hg at 48 months (5.7%) than with a systolic blood pressure below 140 mm Hg at 48 months (4.1%). This study reassures us that hypertensive diabetics treated to a systolic blood pressure goal of below 120 mm Hg will not have a higher prevalence or incidence of orthostatic hypotension than hypertensive diabetics treated to a systolic blood pressure goal below 140 mm Hg [5, 23]. This study also showed that orthostatic hypotension was significantly associated with increased all-cause mortality by 1.62 times and with heart failure death or hospitalization by 1.85 times but not with nonfatal myocardial infarction, stroke, cardiovascular death, or their composite [23].

The Atherosclerosis Risk in Communities study included 12,433 community-dwelling black and white middle-aged men and women, mean age 54 years (57% women and 28% black) [40]. Orthostatic hypotension was present in 5% in this study. At 6-year follow-up, orthostatic hypotension was significantly associated with coronary heart disease by 1.85 times [40]. At 7.9-year follow-up of 11,707 participants free of stroke and clinical heart disease at baseline in the Atherosclerosis Risk in Communities study, orthostatic hypotension was significantly associated with ischemic stroke by 2.0 times [41]. At 17.5-year follow-up of 12,363 persons free of heart failure at baseline in the Atherosclerosis Risk in Communities study, orthostatic hypotension was significantly associated with heart failure by 1.54 times [42]. This association was similar across race and sex groups but was increased 1.90 times in persons aged 55 years and younger and increased 1.37 times in persons older than 55 years [42]. Orthostatic hypotension was present in 76 of 103 new patients (74%) attending a clinic on falls and syncope [43]. A sustained reduction in systolic blood pressure of 30 seconds or longer was associated with a significant increased use of vasopressors by 36% and a significant increased risk of all-cause mortality at 5 years by 45% [43].

A meta-analysis of cardiovascular events and mortality associated with orthostatic hypotension included 13 prospective studies with 121,913 persons [44]. At 5-year follow-up of 65,174 persons, orthostatic hypotension significantly increased all-cause mortality by 1.5 times. At 6.4-year follow-up of 49,512 persons, orthostatic hypotension significantly increased coronary heart disease by 1.41 times. At 6.8 to 24-year follow-up of 50,096 persons, orthostatic hypotension significantly increased heart failure by 2.25 times. At 6.8-year follow-up of 58,300 persons, orthostatic hypotension significantly increased stroke by 1.64 times [44].

A meta-analysis of 8 published papers from 7 cohorts included 64, 782 participants [45]. At 15.2-year follow-up, orthostatic hypotension was associated with a significant increased risk for coronary heart disease by 32% and for stroke by 19% independent of conventional risk factors. This association was significant for both middle-aged and older participants [45]. A meta-analysis of 4 prospective cohort studies which included 51,270 participants and 3603 incident heart failure cases showed that orthostatic hypotension was significantly associated with an increased risk for heart failure by 30% [46].

Treatment

Hypertension should be treated [2]. Persons who have orthostatic hypotension should avoid immobilization, prolonged diurnal recumbence, and physical deconditioning [3, 10, 47, 48]. They should also avoid large meals, isometric exercise, hot weather, hot showers, rapid ascent to a high altitude, hyperventilation, standing motionless, ingesting alcohol, straining at defecation or voiding, diet pills, vasodilators, diuretics, beta agonists, and tricyclic antidepressants. They should gradually rise from the supine and sitting positions, especially in the morning, after meals, and after defecation and urination. Meals should be small. Sodium and water intake should be increased for volume expansion unless heart failure is present. The head of the patient's bed should be raised to a 10°–30° angle during sleep to reduce nocturia, volume depletion, and supine hypertension. Elastic stockings and abdominal compression bandages are recommended to reduce peripheral pooling in the lower limbs and splanchnic region [3, 10, 47–49].

Pharmacological interventions include the direct alpha 1-adrenoreceptor agonist midodrine 2.5 to 10 mg 2 or 3 times daily [47, 48, 50]. The norepinephrine precursor droxidopa 100 to 600 mg 3 times a day may be used [48]. The acetylcholinesterase inhibitor pyridostigmine 30 to 60 mg 2 or 3 times daily is generally recommended only for neurogenic orthostatic hypotension [48]. The mineralocorticoid volume expander fludrocortisone 0.05 to 0.3 mg daily may be used [47, 48]. The efficacy of the direct and indirect alpha 1-adrenoreceptor agonist ephedrine/pseudoephedrine 25/30 to 50/60 mg 3 times daily is controversial [47, 48]. The efficacy of the vasopressin analogue volume expander desmopressin (nasal spray 5 to 40 micrograms daily; oral formulation 100 to 800 micrograms daily) which increases water reabsorption and decreases nocturia is uncertain [48].

Conflict of Interest The author has no conflicts of interest.

References

1. Aronow WS, Lee NH, Sales FF, Etienne F. Prevalence of postural hypotension in elderly patients in a long-term health care facility. Am J Cardiol. 1988;62:336.
2. Aronow WS, Fleg JL, Pepine CJ, et al. ACCF/AHA 2011 expert consensus document on hypertension in the elderly: a report of the American College of Cardiology Foundation Task Force on Clinical Expert Consensus Documents. Developed in collaboration with the American Academy of Neurology, American Geriatrics Society, American Society for Preventive Cardiology, American Society of Hypertension, American Society of Nephrology, Association of Black Cardiologists, and European Society of Hypertension. J Am Coll Cardiol. 2011;57:2037–114.
3. Sciater A, Alagiakrishnan K. Orthostatic hypotension. A primary care primer for assessment and treatment. Geriatrics. 2004;59:22–7.
4. Alagiakrishnan K, Patel K, Desai RV, et al. Orthostatic hypotension and incident heart failure in community-dwelling older adults. J Gerontol Med Sci. 2014;69:223–30.
5. Aronow WS. Orthostatic hypotension in diabetics in the ACCORD (Action to Control Cardiovascular Risk in Diabetes) blood pressure trial. Hypertension. 2016;68:851–2.

6. Aronow WS, Ahn C. Postprandial hypotension in 499 elderly persons in a long-term health care facility. J Am Geriatr Soc. 1994;42:930–2.
7. Aronow WS, Ahn C. Association of postprandial hypotension with incidence of falls, syncope, coronary events, stroke, and total mortality at 29-month follow-up in 499 older nursing home residents. J Am Geriatr Soc. 1997;45:1051–3.
8. Applegate WB, Davis BR, Black HR, et al. Prevalence of postural hypotension at baseline in the Systolic Hypertension in the Elderly Program (SHEP) cohort. J Am Geriatr Soc. 1991;39:1057–64.
9. Maurer M, Rivadeneira H, Bloomfield D. Should orthostatic changes be measured after one or three minutes in elderly subjects? Am Geriatr Cardiol. 1998;7:29–33.
10. Aronow WS. Dizziness and syncope. In: Hazzard WR, Blass JP, Ettinger Jr WH, Halter JB, Ouslander JG, editors. Principles of geriatric medicine and gerontology. 4th ed. McGraw-Hill Inc: New York City; 1999. p. 1519–34.
11. Slavachevsky I, Rachmani R, Levi Z, et al. Effect of enalapril and nifedipine on orthostatic hypotension in older hypertensive patients. J Am Geriatr Soc. 2000;48:807–10.
12. Fan XH, Wang H, Gao LG, et al. The association of an adenine insertion variant in the 5'UTR of the endothelin-1 gene with hypertension and orthostatic hypotension. Arch Med Sci. 2012;8:219–26.. s
13. Lipsitz LA. Orthostatic hypotension in the elderly. N Engl J Med. 1989;321:951–7.
14. Robbins AS, Rubenstein LZ. Postural hypotension in the elderly. J Am Geriatr Soc. 1984;32:769–74.
15. Aronow WS. Effects of aging on the heart. In: Tallis RC, Fillit HM, editors. Brocklehurst's textbook of geriatric medicine and gerontology. 6th ed. London: Churchill Livingstone; 2003. p. 341–8.
16. Gottdiener JS, Yanez D, Rautaharju P, et al. Orthostatic hypotension in the elderly: contributions of impaired LV filling and altered sympathovagal balance. Am J Geriatr Cardiol. 2000;9:273–80.
17. Narkiewicz K, Cooley RL, Somers VK. Alcohol potentiates orthostatic hypotension. Implications for alcohol-related syncope. Circulation. 2000;101:398–402.
18. Finucane C, O'Connell MDL, Fan CW, et al. Age-related normative changes in phasic orthostatic blood pressure in a large population study. Findings from the Irish longitudinal study on ageing (TILDA). Circulation. 2004;130:1780–9.
19. Magnusson M, Holm H, Bachus E, et al. Orthostatic hypotension and cardiac changes after long-term follow-up. Am J Hypertens. 2016;29:847–52.
20. Ferrara LA, Cicerano U, Marotta T, et al. Postprandial and postural hypotension in the elderly. Cardiol Elderly. 1993;1:33–7.
21. Johnson RH, Smith AC, Spalding JMK, et al. Effect of posture on blood pressure in elderly patients. Lancet. 1965;1:731.
22. MacLennan WJ, Hall MRP, Timothy JL. Postural hypotension in old age. Is it a disorder of the nervous system or of blood vessels? Age Ageing. 1980;9:25–32.
23. Fleg JL, Evans GW, Margolis KL, et al. Orthostatic hypotension in the ACCORD (action to control cardiovascular risk in diabetes) blood pressure trial: prevalence, incidence, and prognostic significance. Hypertension. 2016;68:888–95.
24. Wright JT Jr, Williamson JD, Whelton PK, et al. A randomized trial of intensive versus standard blood-pressure control. N Engl J Med. 2015;373:2303–16.
25. Williamson JD, Supiano MA, Applegate WB, et al. Intensive vs standard blood pressure control and cardiovascular disease outcomes in adults aged ≥75 years. A randomized clinical trial. JAMA. 2016;315:2673–82.
26. Tilvis RS, Hakala S-M, Valvanne J, Erkinjuntti T. Postural hypotension and dizziness in a general aged population: a four-year follow-up of the Helsinki aging study. J Am Geriatr. 1996;44:809–14.
27. Weatherford W. The relationship of orthostatic and postprandial hypotension to syncope. Clin Geriatr. 1996;4:58–81.

28. Wu J-S, Lu F-H, Yang Y-C, Chang C-J. Postural hypotension and postural dizziness in patients with non-insulin-dependent diabetes. Arch Intern Med. 1999;159:1350–6.
29. Shaw BH, Loughin TM, Robinovitch SN, Claydon VE. Cardiovascular responses to orthostasic and their association with falls in older adults. BMC Geriatr. 2015;15:174. https://doi.org/10.1186/s12877-015-0168-z.
30. Lilian CM, Pel-Little RE, Jansen PAF, Jansen RWMM. High prevalence of postprandial and orthostatic hypotension among geriatric patients admitted to Dutch hospitals. J Gerontol Med Sci. 2005.; 60A:1271–7.
31. Sule S, Palaniswamy C, Aronow WS, et al. Etiology of syncope in patients hospitalized with syncope and predictors of mortality and readmission for syncope at 17-month follow-up: a prospective study. Am J Ther. 2016;23:e2–6.
32. Palaniswamy C, Aronow WS, Agrawal N, et al. Syncope: approaches to diagnosis and management. Am J Ther. 2016;23:e208–17.
33. Lipsitz LA. Ortostatic hypotension and falls. J Am Geriatr Soc. 2017;65:470–1.
34. Finucane C, O'Connell MDL, Donoghue O, et al. Impaired orthostatic blood pressure recovery is associated with unexplained and injurious falls. J Am Geriatr Soc. 2017;65:474–82.
35. Khera S, Palaniswamy C, Aronow WS, et al. Predictors of mortality, rehospitalization for syncope, and cardiac syncope in 352 consecutive elderly patients with syncope. J Am Med Dir Assoc. 2013;14:326–30.
36. Juraschek SP, Daya N, Rawlings AM, et al. Association of history of dizziness and long-term adverse outcomes with early vs later orthostatic hypotension assessment times in middle-aged adults. JAMA Intern Med. 2017;. PMID 28738139 https://doi.org/10.1001/jamaintern med.2017.2937;177:1316.
37. Masaki KH, Schatz IJ, Burchfiel CM, et al. Orthostatic hypotension predicts mortality in elderly men. The Honolulu Heart Program. Circulation. 1998;98:2290–5.
38. Veronese N, De Rui M, Bolzetta F, et al. Orthostatic changes in blood pressure and mortality in the elderly: the Pro. V. A study. Am J Hypertens. 2015;28:1248–56.
39. Fedorowski A, Stavenow L, Hedblad B, et al. Orthostatic hypotension predicts all-cause mortality and coronary events in middle-aged individuals (the Malmo preventive project). Eur Heart J. 2010;31:85–91.
40. Rose KM, Tyroler HA, Nardo CJ, et al. Orthostatic hypotension and the incidence of coronary heart disease: the atherosclerosis risk in communities study. Am J Hypertens. 2000;13:571–8.
41. Eigenbrodt ML, Rose KM, Couper DJ, et al. Orthostatic hypotension as a risk factor for stroke. The atherosclerosis risk in communities (ARIC) study, 1987–1996. Stroke. 2000;31:2307–13.
42. Jones CD, Loehr L, Franceschini N, et al. Orthostatic hypotension as a risk factor for incident heart failure. The atherosclerosis risk in communities study. Hypertension. 2012;59:913–8.
43. Frith J, Bashir AS, Newton JL. The duration of the orthostatic blood pressure drop is predictive of death. QJM. 2016;109:231–5.
44. Ricci F, Fedorowski A, Radico F, et al. Cardiovascular morbidity and mortality related to orthostatic hypotension: a meta-analysis of prospective observational studies. Eur Heart J. 2015;36:1609–17.
45. Xin W, Mi S, Lin Z, et al. Orthostatic hypotension and the risk of incidental cardiovascular diseases: a meta-analysis of prospective cohort studies. Prev Med. 2016;85:90–7.
46. Xin W, Lin Z, Li X. Orthostatic hypotension and the risk of congestive heart failure: a meta-analysis of prospective cohort studies. PLoS One. 2013;8:e63169.
47. Frishman WH, Azer V, Sica D. Drug treatment of orthostatic hypotension and vasovagal syncope. Heart Dis. 2003;5:49–64.
48. Ricci F, De Caterina R, Fedorowski A. Orthostatic hypotension. Epidemiology, prognosis, and treatment. J Am Coll Cardiol. 2015;66:848–60.
49. Podoleanu C, Maggi R, Brignole M, et al. Lower limb and abdominal compression bandages prevent progressive orthostatic hypotension in elderly persons. A randomized single-blind controlled study. J Am Coll Cardiol. 2006;48:1425–32.
50. Izcovich A, Gonzalez Malla C, Manzotti M, et al. Midodrine for orthostatic hypotension and recurrent reflex syncope: a systematic review. Neurology. 2014;83:1170–7.

Postprandial Hypotension

2

Kannayiram Alagiakrishnan and Darren Mah

Introduction

Postprandial hypotension (PPH) is a significant drop in blood pressure after eating. It is commonly defined as a supine systolic blood pressure (SBP) drop of 20 mmHg or a SBP decrease to less than 90 mmHg when the preprandial SBP is greater than 100 mmHg, within 2 hours of eating [1–3]. In hypertensive subjects, one study showed the cut-off for PPH may be better defined as a SBP drop of 30 mmHg within 2 hours of eating, instead of 20 mmHg [4]. However, there is no standardized definition of PPH. Although orthostatic hypotension (OH) is a common fall concern in the elderly, PPH occurs more often than OH [5].

Epidemiology

PPH is seen in 13% of healthy older adults [6, 7]. Its prevalence increases with certain diseases like diabetes, Parkinson's disease, and chronic renal failure [6, 8–10]. Its prevalence also appears to be increased in patients admitted to the ICU, even after discharge. One small study reported that 29% of patients 65 years or older had PPH 3 months after a stay in an ICU, with an average systolic drop of 10 mmHg among all discharged patients [11]. A study of 85 frail hospitalized older adults found that 67% had PPH compared to 52% with OH [12]. In nursing home subjects, the prevalence of PPH ranges from 24% to 36% [13, 14].

K. Alagiakrishnan (✉)
Division of Geriatric Medicine, University of Alberta, Edmonton, AB, Canada

D. Mah
University of Alberta, Edmonton, AB, Canada

© Springer Nature Switzerland AG 2020
K. Alagiakrishnan, M. Banach (eds.), *Hypotensive Syndromes in Geriatric Patients*, https://doi.org/10.1007/978-3-030-30332-7_2

Causes

PPH is common in elderly patients with autonomic system dysfunction [15]. It occurs in roughly 1/3 of patients with diabetes mellitus [16] and the majority of patients with Parkinson's disease (PD) [17–19]. It is also seen in patients with paraplegia [20, 21] and Alzheimer's disease [22]. Patients with heart failure [23] and hypertension have also been noted to have postprandial blood pressure drops [24–26]. Diuretics like furosemide can potentiate the postprandial blood pressure drop [27].

Pathophysiology

The pathophysiology of PPH is multifactorial (Fig. 2.1). Insulin-induced vasodilation and/or increased postprandial splanchnic blood pooling is an important mechanism [28, 29]. Other factors appear to be impairments in baroreflex function and inadequate postprandial cardiac output increases, peripheral vasoconstriction, and sympathetic nervous system compensation [2, 30]. Reduced baroreflex sensitivity is seen with decreased heart rate variability in PPH [31, 32]. Attenuation of the gastro-vascular reflex plays a role in the mechanism of PPH [33]. In healthy older subjects, postprandial hypotension is associated with relatively more rapid gastric emptying and attenuation of the rise in plasma noradrenaline levels in response to a meal [7, 34]. However, PPH is not fully explained by autonomic dysfunction alone [35]. A

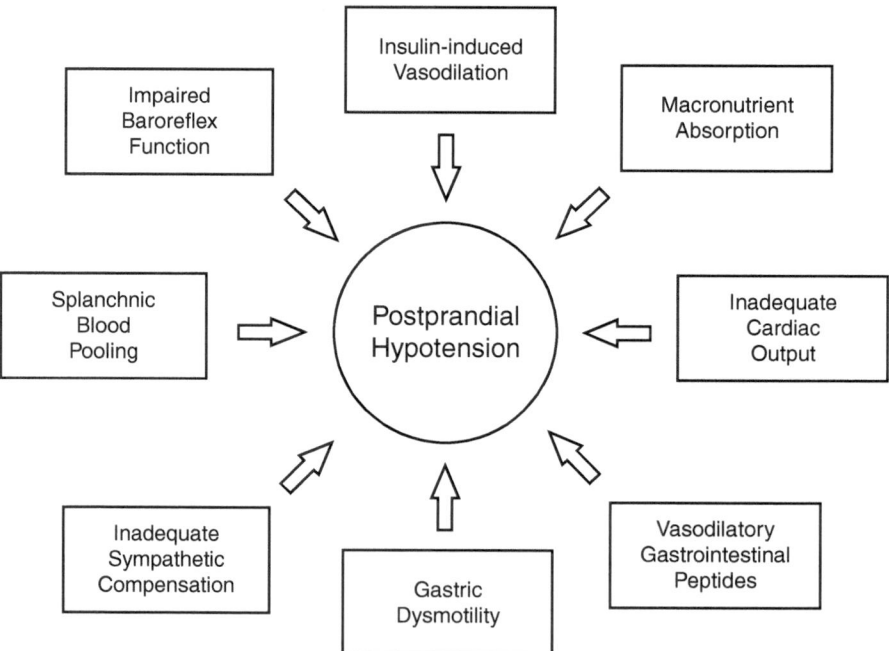

Fig. 2.1 Pathophysiological mechanisms of PPH

number of other mechanisms may also play a role in the pathophysiology of PPH. It may also occur through one or more of the following hormonal mechanisms: release of vasodilatory peptides in the gastrointestinal tract like glucagon-like peptide, vasoactive intestinal peptide, and calcitonin gene-related peptide and/or the release of other hormones like bradykinin, substance P, and neurotensin [36–39].

Gastric distension plays a role in the mechanism of PPH. Gastric distension with water even at low volumes (300 mL) protects the postprandial drop in BP and helps to attenuate PPH [40, 41]. A modest slowing of gastric emptying occurs with healthy aging [42]. Gastroparesis (delayed gastric emptying) occurs commonly with type 2 diabetes mellitus [43], multiple system atrophy (MSA), and PD [44]. The nutrient composition of meals, especially carbohydrates, affects the magnitude of the drop in BP with PPH [41, 45, 46]. In critically ill patients, cardiovascular autonomic dysfunction and gastric dysmotility are more prevalent and may contribute to postprandial hypotension in these subjects [47, 48].

Diagnosis

Due to the general lack of symptoms, PPH is generally underdiagnosed in adults. Barochiner et al. showed home blood pressure monitoring can be used to evaluate PPH [49]. Ambulatory blood pressure monitoring has been used to detect PPH and its clinical implications [50]. Syncope and falls have been correlated with greater post-meal decline in blood pressure using continuous ambulatory blood pressure monitoring [51]. Puisieux et al. in their study of 50 elderly subjects showed the intra-individual reproducibility of PPH was good if the measurements were taken at the same time each day (kappa coefficient = 0.6), but its reproducibility was poor when morning test results were compared with the afternoon test results (kappa coefficient = 0.1) [52].

A simple and quick screening test may help with the diagnosis of PPH, as the current gold standard of measurement requires a 2-hour examination and numerous blood pressure measurements. Abbas et al., after examining 104 patients in geriatric rehabilitation units, suggest that measuring blood pressure before eating and again after 75 minutes may be used to screen patients, with a sensitivity of 82% and specificity of 91% if a cut-off of a drop of 10 mmHg is used. This screening test requires extensive and more comprehensive studies to establish it as a screening test, and to see if other cut-offs and post-meal times would establish better sensitivity without sacrificing specificity [53].

Clinical Presentations

Patients with PPH are often asymptomatic. In one study, Vloet et al. noted that 66% of the study's subjects with PPH were asymptomatic [54]. However, concerning signs and symptoms include dizziness, syncope, falls, and anginal chest pain. Other symptoms include sleepiness, nausea, and headache. Cerebral symptoms depend on the extent to which cerebral perfusion is compromised and the timing of hypotension in PPH. They are also at risk of developing asymptomatic cerebral ischemia, regardless of baseline blood pressure [55, 56]. Patients treated with anti-hypertensives are also at an increased risk of developing PPH. If PPH is due to autonomic dysfunction, reduced appreciation for ischemic events manifesting as chest pain or neurological symptoms can impair timely recognition of ischemia or infarction, thereby delaying appropriate therapy.

Morbidity

A study examined eight older adults with unexplained syncope and found four (50%) had PPH [5]. In another study of patients aged 80–90 years old, PPH was significantly higher in the syncope/falls group than in the control group (23% vs. 9%, $p = 0.03$) [57]. At the same time, PPH is a risk factor for stroke in patients with occlusive cerebrovascular disease and silent lacunar infarcts [55, 58].

Mortality

PPH is an independent predictor of all-cause mortality [59]. This increased mortality appears to not depend on the severity of PPH symptoms. In a prospective study, breakfast-induced PPH has been shown as a possible new risk factor for cardiovascular mortality (HR 1.020, 95% CI 1.001–1.040, $p = 0.04$) [60].

Differential Diagnosis

1. Postprandial hypoglycemia: Patients with postprandial hypoglycemia have a low blood sugar after a meal, usually within 2–4 hours after eating, otherwise known as reactive hypoglycemia. Symptoms include weakness, sweating, and light headedness [61].
2. Orthostatic hypotension (OH): OH is a relatively short-lived phenomenon when compared to PPH, but it is important to note that these conditions can occur together and have additive effects. Vloet et al. showed PPH and OH are more common in geriatric patients than was previously appreciated [62] and can occur due to autonomic dysfunction [63]. PPH is more commonly seen than OH [64].

Management

Management of postprandial hypotension includes a combination of pharmacologic and non- pharmacologic interventions [2] (Table 2.1).

Table 2.1 Non-pharmacological and pharmacological management of postprandial hypotension

Non-pharmacological management	
Patient education – risk of falling after meals	
Supine position postprandially	
Avoid alcohol with meals	
Ensure adequate hydration with eating	
Frequent small meals	
Decrease carbohydrate content in meals	
Drink caffeinated beverages with meals	
Intermittent walking after meals	
Pharmacological management	
Caffeine	250 mg PO, 30 min before meal
Octreotide	25–50 mcg SC, 30 min before meal
Acarbose	25–100 mg PO, 30 min before meal
Voglibose	0.2–0.5 mg PO, 30 min before meal
Guar gum	9 g once daily
Sitagliptin	25 mg every morning

Non-pharmacological

Effective treatment options are presently scarce and relatively limited. Some management approaches that have been tried to date include:

1. Education regarding the risk of falling 15–90 minutes after eating.
2. Remaining in a supine position following a meal.
3. Avoiding alcoholic beverages with large meals [15, 65].
4. Ensuring adequate hydration with eating [41, 66].
5. Encouraging frequent small meals instead of infrequent large meals.
6. Decreasing the amount of carbohydrates in a meal and serving at colder temperatures [67, 68].
7. Coffee drinking with a meal [70].
8. Exercise and walking after meals.

Eating meals with lower amounts of carbohydrates resulted in a smaller decreased duration and magnitude of blood pressure drop in a study of 12 patients with known PPH [69].

A small study has shown that mild exercise after eating in the form of intermittent walking decreased the drop in blood pressure in patients with PPH [71]. At the same time, another study has reported greater drops in blood pressure after supine exercise instead of attenuation. These differences indicate that the type of exercise plays an important role in its effect on blood pressure [72].

Pharmacological

Pharmacological management of PPH based on efficacy and tolerability evidence in the literature has been discussed [73].

Caffeine

Although not completely understood, a proposed mechanism for the effect of caffeine involves antagonization of vasodilators and stimulation of the sympathetic nervous system. There have been previous clinical recommendations regarding caffeine to decrease or prevent postprandial hypotension, but presently there is currently not enough evidence to establish a strong recommendation. However, if given before eating, it may attenuate the blood pressure drop in some patients. It may be taken in liquid or tablet form. However, no standardized dosing has been established, with reported doses ranging from 60 to 200 mg. Due to the availability of caffeine and caffeine-containing foods, it is worth trying in patients who are affected by PPH. Reported side effects include diarrhea, tremors, and sleep disorders [74, 75].

Octreotide

Octreotide is a treatment for patients with known autonomic failure, and some clinicians have suggested its use be expanded to include patients with PPH. Its proposed mechanism appears to include an increase in splanchnic blood flow and peripheral vascular resistance as well as the antagonization of intestinal and pancreatic hormones. To date, three small studies have shown a significant improvement in reducing postprandial blood pressure drop with octreotide without significant side effects. However, in practice, it is costly to patients and may be inconvenient because it must be administered subcutaneously before meals. Standard doses range from 25 to 50 mcg. Notable potential side effects include pain at the site of injection, nausea, diarrhea, and alopecia [76–78].

Alpha-Glucosidase Inhibitors

Acarbose and voglibose reduce splanchnic blood flow by delaying gastric emptying and intestinal complex carbohydration metabolism, a proposed mechanism by which they decrease postprandial hypotension. Delayed carbohydrate metabolism decreases the secretion of insulin, leading to decreased vasodilation. They have been shown to improve symptoms in the short term, but further long-term efficacy studies have yet to be completed. Acarbose is generally dosed at 100 mg orally 20 minutes preprandially three times per day. Side effects of alpha-glucosidase inhibitors include abdominal pain, diarrhea, and flatulence [79–82].

3,4-DL-Threo-Dihydroxyphenylserine

One 1996 study examined 3,4-DL-threo-dihydroxyphenylserine (DL-DOPS), a norepinephrine precursor, on 11 patients with postprandial hypotension and autonomic failure. DL-DOPS mitigated some of the postprandial drop in hypotension without affecting heart rate. However, to date, there have been no further reported long-term investigations into the use of DL-DOPS or other catecholamine-related therapies in PPH [83].

Guar Gum

Guar gum, a guar bean derivative historically used in the food industry, has been implicated in studies as a potential way to mediate postprandial hypotension. Like alpha-glucosidase inhibitors, a proposed mechanism for its effect includes delayed gastric emptying and intestinal absorption. However, standard dosing regimens for guar gum do not exist, and no long-term studies have examined its efficacy for PPH. Common side effects of guar gum include abdominal pain, diarrhea, and flatulence [84, 85].

Sitagliptin

Sitagliptin, a dipeptidyl peptidase-4 (DPP-4) inhibitor used primarily in the treatment of diabetes mellitus, was reported to have successfully treated a 78-year-old woman with symptomatic postprandial hypotension in a case study. The patient also had known orthostatic hypotension and cognitive impairment, and was later diagnosed with dementia with Lewy bodies. In addition to her PPH, her OH and cognitive impairment also improved with the administration of sitagliptin. A potential mechanism for this improvement is increased GLP-1 activity which stimulates glucose-dependent insulin secretion, attenuates glucagon secretion, and slows gastric emptying. As no large studies other than case reports have been published regarding sitagliptin or other DPP-4 inhibitors and their effect on PPH, more studies with larger cohorts of patients and controls are required to evaluate short- and long-term efficacy [86, 87].

Other Pharmacologic Agents

A number of drugs, including midodrine, fludrocortisone, and vasopressin, have all given variable results in different studies for the management of PPH. However, limitations in study design and power mean that to date there is no strong evidence to suggest their efficacy in patients with PPH [2].

PPH with Chronic Medical Conditions

PPH has been associated with number of chronic medical conditions [88].

PPH and Hypertension

Studies have shown that the occurrence of PPH is increased among individuals with systolic hypertension compared to those without [89, 90]. In essential hypertensive patients, PPH is also associated with asymptomatic cerebrovascular damage and may act as a strong risk factor in patients with known cerebrovascular disease to develop stroke [56].

Patients with symptomatic or severe postprandial hypotension benefit from less stringent blood pressure targets [91]. Adequate treatment of hypertension and avoidance of diuretics and nitrates may help to reduce the postprandial blood pressure drop.

PPH and Diabetes

Autonomic neuropathy secondary to diabetes can lead to PPH. One study estimated the prevalence of PPH in those with type 2 diabetes mellitus (T2DM) to be 30–40%. Additionally, in more than 10% of people with long-term T2DM, PPH and OH occur together [9, 92]. Alpha-glucosidase inhibitors such as acarbose and voglibose, once indicated for the treatment of diabetes itself, have been shown to be helpful to treat PPH in individuals with diabetes [80, 92].

PPH and Neurological Disorders

Due to autonomic dysfunction, PPH is common in patients with neurological disorders such as multiple system atrophy (MSA) and Parkinson's disease (PD). This association was reported in a case study as early as 1977. Recent study has shown some key risk factors for the development of PPH in a population of patients with PD, including constipation, dysosmia, baseline hypertension, and an orthostatic systolic blood pressure drop of greater than 30 mmHg. The risk factors with the highest sensitivity/specificity were constipation, hypertension, and orthostatic systolic blood pressure drop greater than 30 mmHg. Studies to date have not examined if the management of some of these comorbid symptoms in PD may help to change the course of PPH.

In two small Japanese studies looking at PPH in MSA, there was an increased prevalence of PPH. One study reported that all 10 patients with MSA had PPH (100%), whereas the other reported 58% of 24 patients had PPH. Some of this difference may be at least partly attributable to different definitions of PPH; the former study used a cut-off of a drop of 15 mmHg 15 minutes postprandially, whereas the latter used a cut-off of 20 mmHg within 60 minutes [93–97]. PPH can also cause headache, and treatment of PPH relieved headache in a case series [98].

PPH and Syncope, Falls

PPH is more commonly seen in subjects with falls [99]. Regarding morbidity associated with PPH, one study showed that 23% of hospitalized elderly patients with either syncope or falls had PPH [13]. Le Couteur et al. showed that the risk of fall increases in subjects who had a postprandial systolic blood pressure drop below 115 mmHg [100]. In elderly patients at nursing homes, 6–8% of syncopal episodes could be attributed to PPH [101]. In hospitalized subjects with unexplained syncope, Jansen et al. showed half had postprandial hypotension [5].

Conclusions

PPH is a significant fall in blood pressure after food ingestion. Its pathophysiology stems from a number of causes. PPH should be considered in any elderly patient with falls, syncope, dizziness, or cardiac or cerebral ischemic symptoms. Prompt diagnosis and proper management can help decrease the morbidity and mortality seen in elderly subjects with PPH. Increasing awareness of this hypotensive syndrome can lead to decreased falls and syncope and the avoidance of unnecessary testing in these conditions. With patient education, non-pharmacological and pharmacological management, this condition can be adequately addressed in elderly subjects.

References

1. Lipsitz LA, Nyquist RP Jr, Wei JY, et al. Postprandial reduction in blood pressure in the elderly. N Engl J Med. 1983;309:81–3.
2. Jansen RW, Lipsitz LA. Postprandial hypotension: epidemiology, pathophysiology and clinical management. Ann Intern Med. 1995;122:286–95.
3. Luciano GL, Brennan MJ, Rothberg MB. Postprandial hypotension. Am J Med. 2010;123:2811e–6e.
4. Wieling W, Schatz IJ. The consensus statement on the definition of orthostatic hypotension: a revisit after 13 years. J Hypertens. 2009;27(5):935–8.
5. Jansen RW, Connelly CM, Kelly-Gagnon MM, et al. Postprandial hypotension in elderly patients with unexplained syncope. Arch Intern Med. 1995;155:945–52.
6. Trahair LG, Horowitz M, Jones KL. Postprandial hypotension: a systematic review. J Am Med Dir Assoc. 2014;15(6):394–409.
7. Trahair LG, Horowitz M, Jones KL. Postprandial hypotension is associated with more rapid gastric emptying in healthy older individuals. J Am Med Dir Assoc. 2015;16(6):521–3.
8. Trahair LG, Kimber TE, Flabouris K, et al. Gastric emptying, postprandial blood pressure, glycaemia and splanchnic flow in Parkinson's disease. World J Gastroenterol. 2016;22(20):4860–7.
9. Jones KL, Tonkin A, Horowitz M, Wishart JM, Carney BI, Guha S, et al. Rate of gastric emptying is a determinant of postprandial hypotension in non-insulindependent diabetes mellitus. Clin Sci (Lond). 1998;94:65e70.
10. Sherman RA, Torres F, Cody RP. Postprandial blood pressure changes during hemodialysis. Am J Kidney Dis. 1988;12:37e9.
11. Nguyen TAN, Ali Abdelhamid Y, Weinel LM, Hatzinikolas S, Kar P, Summers MJ, Phillips LK, Horowitz M, Jones KL, Deane AM. Postprandial hypotension in older survivors of critical illness. J Crit Care. 2018;45:20–6.
12. Vloet LC, Pel-Little RE, Jansen PA, et al. High prevalence of postprandial and orthostatic hypotension among geriatric patients admitted to Dutch hospitals. J Gerontological A Biol Sci Med Sci. 2005;60:1271–7.
13. Aronow WS, Ahn C. Postprandial hypotension in 499 elderly persons in a long-term healthcare facility. J Am Geriatr Soc. 1994;42:930–2.
14. Vaitkeviclus PV, Esserwein DM, Maynard AK, et al. Frequency and importance of postprandial blood pressure reduction in elderly nursing home patients. Ann Intern Med. 1991;115:865–70.
15. Luciano GL, Brennan MJ, Rothberg MB. Postprandial hypotension. Am J Med. 2010;123:281. e1–6.
16. Sasaki E, Kitaoka H, Ohsawa N. Postprandial hypotension in patients with Non insulin-dependent diabetes mellitus. Diabetes Res Clin Pract. 1992;18:113e121.
17. Micieli G, Martignoni E, Cavallini A, et al. Postprandial and orthostatic hypotension in Parkinson's disease. Neurology. 1987;37:386e393.
18. Loew F, Gauthey L, Koerffy A, et al. Postprandial hypotension and orthostatic blood pressure responses in elderly Parkinson's disease patients. J Hypertens. 1995;13:1291e1297.
19. Chaudhuri KR, Ellis C, Love-Jones S, et al. Postprandial hypotension and parkinsonian state in Parkinson's disease. Mov Disord. 1997;12:877e884.
20. Baliga RR, Catz AB, Watson LD, et al. Cardiovascular and hormonal responses to food ingestion in humans with spinal cord transection. Clin Auton Res. 1997;7:137e141.
21. Catz A, Bluvshtein V, Pinhas I, et al. Hemodynamic effects of liquid food ingestion in mid-thoracic paraplegia: is supine postprandial hypotension related to thoracic spinal cord damage? Spinal Cord. 2007;45:96e103.
22. Idiaquez J, Rios L, Sandoval E. Postprandial hypotension in Alzheimer's disease. Clin Auton Res. 1997;7:119e120.

23. Cornyn JW, Massie BM, Unverferth DV, Leier CV. Hemodynamics changes after meals and placebo treatment in chronic congestive heart failure. Am J Cardio/. 1986;57:238–41.
24. Masuo K, Mikami H, Habara N, Ogihara T. Orthostatic and postprandial blood pressure reduction in patients with essential hypertension. Clin Exp Pharmacol Physiol. 1991;18:155–61.
25. Masuo K, Mikami H, Habara N, Ogihara T. The mechanisms of postprandial blood pressure reduction in elderly patients with essential hypertension. Eur JGerontol. 1993;2:13–9.
26. Jansen RW, Lenders JW, Thien T, Hoefnagels WH. Antihypertensive treatment and postprandial blood pressure reduction in the elderly. Gerontology. 1987;32:363–8.
27. Mitro P, Feterik K, Cverckova A, Trejbal D. Occurrence and relevance of postprandial hypotension in patients with essential hypertension. Wien Klin Wochenschr. 1999;111:320–5.
28. Staneczek O, Abbas-Terki N, Loew F, Sieber CC. A full stomach but an empty head. J Am Geriatr Soc. 2001;49:1262–3.
29. Kearney MT, Cowley AJ, Stubbs TA, et al. Depressor action of insulin on skeletal muscle vasculature: a novel mechanism for postprandial hypotension in the elderly. J Am Coll Cardiol. 1998;31:209–16.
30. Aronow WS, Ahn C. Postprandial hypotension in 499 elderly persons in a long-term health care facility. J Am Geriatr Soc. 1994;42:930–2.
31. Teramoto S, Akishita M, Fukuchi Y, et al. Assessment of autonomic nervous function in elderly subjects with or without postprandial hypotension. Hypertens Res. 1997;20:257–26.
32. Kawaguchi R, Nomura M, Miyajima H, et al. Postprandial hypotension in elderly subjects: spectral analysis of heart rate variability and electrogastrograms. J Gastroenterol. 2002;37:87–93.
33. van Orshoven NP, Oey PL, van Schelven LJ, Roelofs JMM, Jansen PAF, Akkermans LMA. Effect of gastric distension on cardiovascular parameters: gastrovascular reflex is attenuated in the elderly. J Physiol. 2004;555(2):573–83.
34. Tanakaya M, Takahashi N, Takeuchi K, et al. Postprandial hypotension due to a lack of sympathetic compensation in patients with diabetes mellitus. Acta Med Okayama. 2007;61:191–7.
35. Lagro J, Meel-van den Abeelen A, de Jong DL, et al. Geriatric hypotensive syndromes are not explained by cardiovascular autonomic dysfunction alone. J Gerontol A Biol Sci Med Sci. 2012;68:581–9.
36. Mathias CJ, da Costa DF, Fosbraey P, et al. Cardiovascular, biochemical and hormonal changes during food-induced hypotension in chronic autonomic failure. J Neurol Sci. 1989;94:255–69.
37. Bremholm L, Hornum M, Henriksen BM, et al. Glucagon-like peptide-2 increases mesenteric blood flow in humans. Scand J Gastroenterol. 2009;44:314–9.
38. Edwards BJ, Perry HMIII, Kaiser FE, et al. Relationship of age and calcitonin gene-related peptide to postprandial hypotension. Mech Ageing Dev. 1996;87:61–73.
39. Tumilero S, Gallo L, Foss MC, et al. Role of bradykinin in postprandial hypotension in humans. Braz J Med Bio Res. 1999;32:777–81.
40. Gentilcore D, Meyer JH, Rayner CK, et al. Gastric distension attenuates the hypotensive effect of intraduodenal glucose in healthy older subjects. Am J Physiol Regul Integr Comp Physiol. 2008;295:R472–7.
41. Jones KL, O'Donovan D, Russo A, et al. Effects of drink volume and glucose load on gastric emptying and postprandial blood pressure in healthy older subjects. Am J Physiol Gastrointest Liver Physiol. 2005;289:G240–8.
42. Horowitz M, Maddern GJ, Chatterton BE, et al. Changes in gastric emptying rates with age. Clin Sci (Lond). 1984;67:213–8.
43. Jones KL, Tonkin A, Horowitz M, et al. Rate of gastric emptying is a determinant of postprandial hypotension in noninsulin-dependent diabetes mellitus. Clin Sci (Lond). 1998;94:65–70.
44. Thomaides T, Karapanayiotides T, Zoukos Y, et al. Gastric emptying after semisolid food in multiple system atrophy and Parkinson disease. J Neurol. 2005;252:1055–9.
45. Vanis L, Gentilcore D, Hausken T, et al. Effects of gastric distension on blood pressure and superior mesenteric artery blood flow responses to intraduodenal glucose in healthy older subjects. Am J Physiol Regul Integr Comp Physiol. 2010;299:R960–7.

46. Visvanathan R, Horowitz M, Chapman I. The hypotensive response to oral fat is comparable but slower compared with carbohydrate in healthy elderly subjects. Br J Nutr. 2006;95:340–5.
47. Schmidt H, Muller-Werdan U, Hoffmann T, et al. Autonomic dysfunction predicts mortality in patients with multiple organ dysfunction syndrome of different age groups. Crit Care Med. 2005;33(9):1994–2002.
48. Kar P, Jones KL, Horowitz M, et al. Measurement of gastric emptying in the critically ill. Clin Nutr. 2015;34(4):557–64.
49. Barochiner J, Alfie J, Aparicio L, Cuffaro P, Rada M, Morales M, et al. Postprandial hypotension detected through home blood pressure monitoring: a frequent phenomenon in elderly hypertensive patients. Hypertens Res. 2014;37:438–43.
50. Kohara K, Uemura K, Takata Y, et al. Postprandial hypotension: evaluation by ambulatory blood pressure monitoring. Am J Hypertens. 1998;11:1358–63.
51. Puisieux F, Bulckaen H, Fauchais AL, Drumez S, Salomez-Granier F, Dewailly P. Ambulatory blood pressure monitoring and postprandial hypotension in elderly persons with falls or syncopes. J Gerontol A. 2000;55(9):M535–40.
52. Puisieux F, Court D, Baheau F, et al. Intraindividual reproducibility of post-prandial hypotension. Gerontology. 2002;48:315–20.
53. Abbas R, Tanguy A, Bonnet-Zamponi D, Djedid R, Lounis A, Gaubert-Dahan ML. New simplified screening method for postprandial hypotension in older people. J Frailty Aging. 2018;7(1):28–33.
54. Vloet LC, Pel-Littel RE, Jansen PA, Jansen RWMM. High prevalence of postprandial and orthostatic hypotension among geriatric patients admitted to Dutch hospitals. J Gerontol A Biol Sci Med Sci. 2005;60A:1271–7.
55. Tabara Y, Okada Y, Uetani E, Nagai T, Igase M, Kido T, et al. Postprandial hypotension as a risk marker for asymptomatic lacunar infarction. J Hypertens. 2014;32:1084–90.
56. Kohara K, Jiang Y, Igase M, Takata Y, Fukuoka T, Okura T, et al. Postprandial hypotension is associated with asymptomatic cerebrovascular damage in essential hypertensive patients. Hypertension. 1999;33:565–8.
57. Pulsieux F, Bulckaen FAL, et al. Ambulatory blood pressure monitoring and postprandial hypotension in elderly persons with falls or syncopes. J Gerontol A Biol Sci Med Sci. 2000;. 55A;55:M535–40.
58. Aronow WS, Ahn C. Association of postprandial hypotension with incidence of falls, syncope, coronary events, stroke, and total mortality at 29- months follow-up in 499 older nursing home residents. J Am Geriatr Soc. 1997;45:1051–3.
59. Fisher AA, Davis MW, Srikusalanukul W, et al. Postprandial hypotension predicts all- cause mortality in older, low- level care residents. J Am Ger Soc. 2005;53:1313–20.
60. Zanasi A, Tincani E, Evandri V, Giovanardi P, Bertolotti M, Rioli G. Meal induced blood pressure variation and cardiovascular mortality in ambulatory hypertensive elderly patients: preliminary results. J Hypertens. 2012;30:2125–32.
61. Brun JF, Fedou C, Mercier J. Postprandial reactive hypoglycemia. Diabetes Metab. 2000;26:337.
62. Vloet LC, Pel-Little RE, Jansen PA, Jansen RW. High prevalence of postprandial and orthostatic hypotension among geriatric patients admitted to Dutch hospitals. J Gerontol A Biol Sci Med Sci. 2005 Oct;60(10):1271–7.
63. Tamura N. Orthostatic hypotension and postprandial hypotension. Rinsho Shinkeigaku. 1996 Dec;36(12):1349–51.
64. Jansen RWMM, Kelley-Gagnon MM, Lipsitz LA. Intraindividual reproducibility of post-prandial and orthostatic blood pressure changes in older nursing-home patients: relationship with chronic use of cardiovascular medications. J Am Geriatr Soc. 1996;44:383–9.
65. Jansen RW, Hoefnagels WH. Postprandial blood pressure reduction. Neth J Med. 1990;37:80–8.
66. Son JT, Lee E. Effect of water drinking on the postprandial fall of blood pressure in the elderly. J Korean Acad Fundam Nurs. 2010;17(3):304–13.

67. Vloet LC, Smits R, Jansen RW. The effect of meals at different mealtimes on blood pressure and symptoms in geriatric patients with postprandial hypotension. J Gerontol A Biol Sci Med Sci. 2003;58(11):1031–5.
68. Kuipers HM, Jansen RW, Peeters TL, Hoefnalgels WH. The influence of food temperature on postprandial blood pressure reduction and its relation to substance-P in healthy elderly subjects. J Am Geriatr Soc. 1991;39(2):181–4.
69. Vloet LC, Mehagnoul-Schipper DJ, Hoefnagels WHL, Jansen RWMM. The influence of low-, normal-, and high-carbohydrate meals on blood pressure in elderly patients with postprandial hypotension. J Gerontol A Biol Sci Med Sci. 2001.;56A;56:M744–8.
70. Rakic V, Beilin IJ, Burke V. Effect of coffee and tea drinking on postprandial hypotension in older men and women. Clin Exp Pharmacol Physiol. 1996;23:559–63.
71. Nair S, Visvanathan R, Gentilcore D. Intermittent walking: a potential treatment for older people with postprandial hypotension. JAMDA. 2015;16:160e–4e.
72. Puvi-Rajasingham S, Smith GDP, Akinola A, Mathias CJ. Hypotensive and regional haemodyanamic effects of exercise, fasted and after food, in human sympathetic denervation. Clin Sci (Lond). 1998;94:49–55.
73. Alagiakrishnan K. Drugs Aging. 2015;32(5):337–48.
74. Robertson D, Frolich JC, Carr RK, et al. Effects of caffeine on plasma renin activity, catecholamines and blood pressure. N Engl J Med. 1978;298:181–6.
75. Lipsitz LA, Jansen RW, Connelly CM, et al. Haemodynamic and neurohumoral effects of caffeine in elderly patients with symptomatic postprandial hypotension: a double-blind, randomized, placebo-controlled study. Clin Sci (Lond). 1994;87:259–67.
76. Jansen RWMM, Peeters TL, Lenders JWM, et al. Somtostatin analog octreotide (SMS 201–995) prevents the decrease in blood pressure after oral glucose loading in the elderly. J Clin Endocrinol Metab. 1989;68:752–6.
77. Jansen RWMM, Lenders JWM, Peeters TL, et al. SMS 201–995 prevents postprandial blood pressure reduction in normotensive and hypertensive elderly subjects. J Hypertens. 1988;. S6;6:S669–72.
78. Alam M, Smith G, Bleasdale- Barr K, et al. Effects of the peptide release inhibitor, octreotide on daytime hypotension and on nocturnal hypertension in primary autonomic failure. J Hypertens. 1995;13:1664–9.
79. Gentilcore D, Bryant B, Wishart JM, et al. Acarbose attenuates the hypotensive response to sucrose and slows gastric emptying in the elderly. Am J Med. 2005;118:1289.
80. Maruta T, Komai K, Takamori M, Yamada M. Voglibose inhibits postprandial hypotemnsion in neurological disorders and elderly people. Neurology. 2006;66:1432–4.
81. Shibao C, Gamboa A, Diedrich A, et al. Acarbose, an alpha-glucosidase inhibitor attenuates postprandial hypotension in autonomic failure. Hypertension. 2007;50:54–61.
82. Jian ZJ, Zhou BV. Efficacy and safety of acarbose in the treatment of elderly patients with postprandial hypotension. Chin Med J. 2008;121:2054–9.
83. Freeman B, Young J, Landsberg L, Lipsitz L. The treatment of postprandial hypotension in autonomic failure with DL-threo dihydroxy phenyl serine. Neurology. 1996;47:1414–20.
84. Jones KL, Macintosh C, Su YC, Wells F, Chapman IM, Tonkin A, Horowitz M. Guar gum reduces post prandial hypotension in older people. J Am Geriatr Soc. 2001;49(2):162–7.
85. Russo A, Stevens JE, Wilson T, Wells F, Tonkin A, Horowitz M, Jones KL. Guar attenuates fall in postprandial blood pressure and slows gastric emptying of oral glucose in type 2 diabetes. Dig Dis Sci. 2003;48(7):1221–9.
86. Saito Y, Ishikawa J, Harada K. Postprandial and orthostatic hypotension treated by Sitagliptin in a patient with dementia with Lewy bodies. Am J Case Rep. 2016;17:887–93.
87. Yonenaga A, Ota H, Honda M, et al. Marked improvement of elderly postprandial hypotension by dipeptidyl peptidase IV inhibitor. Geriatr Gerontol Int. 2013;13:227–9.
88. Alagiakrishnan K. Postural and postprandial hypotension: approach to management. Geriatr Aging. 2007;10(5):298–304.
89. Mitro P, Feterik K, Cverckova A, et al. Occurrence and relevance of postprandial hypotension in patients with essential hypertension. Wien Klin Wochenschr. 1999;111:320–5.

90. Grodzicki T, Rajzer M, Fagard R, et al. Ambulatory blood pressure monitoring and postprandial hypotension in elderly patients with isolated systolic hypertension. J Hum Hypertens. 1998;12:161–5.
91. Alfie J. Utility of home blood pressure monitoring to evaluate postprandial blood pressure in treated hypertensive patients. Ther Adv Cardiovasc Dis. 2015;9(4):133–9.
92. Sasaki E, Goda K, Nagata K, et al. Acarbose improved severe postprandial hypotension in patient with diabetes mellitus. J Diabetes Complicat. 2001;15:158–61.
93. Loew F, Gauthey L, Koerffy A, Herrmann FR, Estade M, Michel JP, et al. Postprandial hypotension and orthostatic blood pressure responses in elderly Parkinson's disease patients. J Hypertens. 1995;13:1291e7.
94. Chaudhuri KR, Ellis C, Love-Jones S, Thomaides T, Clift S, Mathias CJ, et al. Postprandial hypotension and parkinsonian state in Parkinson's disease. Mov Disord. 1997;12:877–84.
95. Umehara T, Nakahara A, Matsuno H, Toyoda C, Oka H. Predictors of postprandial hypotension in elderly patients with de novo Parkinson's disease. J Neural Transm (Vienna). 2016;123(11):1331–9.
96. Fukushima T, Asahina M, Fujinuma Y, et al. Role of intestinal peptides and the autonomic nervous system in post prandial hypotension in patients with multiple system atrophy. J Neurol. 2012;260:475–81.
97. https://doi.org/10.1016/0165-1838(93)90315-L.
98. Tazikawa T, Shibata M, Hiraide T. Possible involvement of hypotension in postprandial headache: a case series. Headache. 2017;57:1443–8.
99. Maurer MS, Karmally W, Rivadeneira H, Parides MK, Bloomfield DM. Upright posture and postprandial hypotension in elderly persons. Ann Intern Med. 2000;133:533–6.
100. Le Couteur DG, Fisher AA, Davis MW, McLean AJ. Postprandial systolic blood pressure responses of older people in residential care: association with risk of falling. Gerontology. 2003;49:260–4.
101. Lipsitz LA, Pluchino FC, Wie JY, Rowe JW. Syncope in institutionalized elderly: the impact of multiple pathological conditions and situational stress. J Chronic Dis. 1986;39:619–30.

Carotid Sinus Syndrome

Anna Kasperowicz, Maciej Banach, Marek Maciejewski, and Agata Bielecka-Dabrowa

History

First reports concerning the slowing of heart rate as a result of pressure on a carotid artery can be found already in the publication of Parry from 1799 [1]. In 1866, Czermak documented a drop in blood pressure as a response to a pressure on (own) carotid artery [2]. The term 'carotid sinus hypersensitivity' (CSH) was used for the first time in 1930 by Roskan [3] in order to describe the phenomenon of asystole with the loss of consciousness in response to pressure on a carotid artery. The relationship between the stimulation of carotid sinus and spontaneous syncope was described by Weiss and Baker in 1933 [4]. The origins of the definition of carotid sinus hypersensitivity in the form of cardiodepression (asystole for at least 3 seconds [s]) can be found in the work of these two researchers. In 1946, Nathanson [5], for the first time, distinguished between carotid sinus syndrome (CSS) leading to syncope triggered by the stimulation of carotid sinus associated with daily activities and carotid sinus hypersensitivity (CSH). In the 1960s, Franke defined the criteria for the vasodepressor form of CSH [6]. At the beginning of the twenty-first century, Kerr [7] and Krediet [8] proposed modified, stricter criteria for the diagnosis of carotid sinus syndrome. In a review from 2013, Wieling and colleagues postulate

A. Kasperowicz
University Hospital, Clinical Department of Cardiology, Zielona Gora, Poland

M. Banach · A. Bielecka-Dabrowa (✉)
Department of Hypertension, Chair of Nephrology and Hypertension,
Medical University of Lodz, Lodz, Poland

Department of Cardiology and Congenital Diseases of Adults,
Polish Mother's Memorial Hospital Research Institute (PMMHRI), Lodz, Poland
e-mail: agata.bielecka-dabrowa@iczmp.edu.pl

M. Maciejewski
Department of Cardiology and Congenital Diseases of Adults,
Polish Mother's Memorial Hospital Research Institute (PMMHRI), Lodz, Poland

© Springer Nature Switzerland AG 2020
K. Alagiakrishnan, M. Banach (eds.), *Hypotensive Syndromes in Geriatric Patients*, https://doi.org/10.1007/978-3-030-30332-7_3

that all patients should be thought of as having multiple forms of hypersensitivity: cardio- and vasodepressor with various dominant mechanisms [9]. According to the guidelines of the European Society of Cardiology (ESC) on the diagnosis and management of synapse of 2018, carotid sinus hypersensitivity is defined as an asystole lasting at least 3 s and/or a pressure fall by more than 50 mmHg [10].

The Carotid Artery Sinus

The carotid artery sinus is located in the upper part of the common carotid artery just below the division into the internal and external carotid arteries. Numerous baro- and mechanoreceptors are located within its wall. These receptors are the endings of vascular fibres of vagus nerve fibres and laryngopharyngeal nerves. Under the influence of blood pressure changes or a pressure on the carotid sinus, the receptors transmit impulses to a vagal nerve nucleus and a vasomotor centre in the brain stem. Further, these impulses are transmitted via vagus nerve fibres to a sinoatrial node and atrioventricular node and via sympathetic fibres to the heart and blood vessels.

Receptor stimulation results in the triggering of a reflex in the form of heart rate slowing, decrease in contractility, vasodilatation, and, as a result, a fall in blood pressure.

Decreased activity of baroreceptors results in vasoconstriction and the acceleration of cardiac function [9, 11].

Carotid Sinus Syndrome and Carotid Sinus Hypersensitivity: Epidemiology and Diagnosis

Carotid sinus syndrome (CSS) is a disease of an autonomic nervous system, in which a hypersensitivity of carotid sinus receptors occurs. Main symptoms of this syndrome involve spontaneous syncope caused by unintentional pressure on the carotid artery sinus (e.g. when shaving or tying a tie) [8]. The CSS syndrome is rare; it is observed in c.a. 1% of patients with documented syncope [9], mainly in older people (~75 years old). In men, it is over two times as prevalent as in women [12]. It is estimated that the incidence of CSS in patients admitted to specialized centres due to fainting is less than 4% in persons under the age of 40 years, but it reaches 41% in patients over 80 years [13, 14].

The diagnosis of CSS is based on the history of syncope and a positive result of carotid sinus massage test. This test is considered as positive when a syncope occurs during a 10-s massage or immediately after its completion as a result of cardioinhibitory or vasodepressive reaction. CSS can be triggered by a pressure on the carotid sinus, e.g. by an additional neck rib, by a tight shirt collar or a tumour. Other causes include a sharp increase in pressure in the common carotid artery coexisting with cough or physical exertion. Patients with CSS and a past history of syncope or loss of consciousness usually have no presyncope symptoms. At the same time, these patients often suffer severe injuries or fractures [15]. Carotid sinus hypersensitivity (CSH) is a related condition where CSM is positive in an asymptomatic patient. Carotid sinus hypersensitivity in patients with unexplained syncope may be a non-specific finding because it is present in <40% of older populations and should be used with caution for diagnosis of the mechanism of syncope. CSH cannot be assumed to respond to pacing. The incidence of this syndrome is estimated to be 26–60% [9]. The pathophysiology of CSH is complex, and some of its aspects are not fully understood. Early diagnosis and appropriate treatment of this condition may improve morbidity and prevent complications in elderly people [16]. CSH is common in patients with neurodegenerative disorders and dementia [17].

CSS and CSH are closely related. In accordance with the current guidelines of the European Society of Cardiology on the diagnosis and the management of syncope, CSH is diagnosed in patients in whom CSM induces asystole lasting for at least 3 s or a decrease in systolic blood pressure by at least 50 mmHg or both [8, 10]. Classification of CSS after CSM with and without usage of atropine based on Brignole and Menozzi was presented in Table 3.1 [18]. It should be underlined that according to ESC guidelines of 2018, in certain cases [9], the asystole may last over 6 s [10].

Vasodepressive type (VDCSH) in which a pressure fall by more than 50 mmHg in comparison to baseline pressure is observed.

Carotid sinus hypersensitivity (CSH) is a related condition where CSM is positive in an asymptomatic patient. Carotid sinus hypersensitivity in patients with unexplained syncope may be a non-specific finding because it is present in <40% of older populations and should be used with caution for diagnosis of the mechanism of syncope. CSH cannot be assumed to respond to pacing. The incidence of this syndrome is estimated to be 26–60% [9]. The pathophysiology of CSH is complex, and some of its aspects are not fully understood. Early diagnosis and appropriate treatment of this condition may improve morbidity and prevent complications in elderly people [16]. CSH is common in patients with neurodegenerative disorders and dementia [17].

Table 3.1 Classification of CSS (Based on Brignole and Menozzi) [18]

Classification of CSS		
Dominant cardioinhibitory CSS	Mixed CSS	Dominant vasodepressor CSS
Initial CSM		
Ventricular asystole >3 s + reproduction of spontaneous symptoms.	Ventricular asystole >3 s + reproduction of spontaneous symptoms.	Ventricular asystole absent or < 3 s + BP fall >50 mmHg with reproduction of spontaneous symptoms.
CSM + atropine		
Absence of ventricular asystole and symptoms (vasodepressor component either insufficient to cause symptoms or absent).	BP fall >50 mmHg with reproduction of spontaneous symptoms.	Ventricular asystole absent, BP fall as with initial CSM + reproduction of spontaneous symptoms.

CSS carotid sinus syndrome, *CSM* carotid sinus massage, *BP* blood pressure. Atropine administered IV 0.02 mg/kg body weight.

CSS and CSH are closely related. In accordance with the current guidelines of the European Society of Cardiology on the diagnosis and the management of syncope, CSH is diagnosed in patients in whom CSM induces asystole lasting for at least 3 s or a decrease in systolic blood pressure by at least 50 mmHg or both [8, 10]. It should be underlined that according to ESC guidelines of 2018, in certain cases [9], the asystole may last over 6 s [10].

On the basis of the aforementioned assumptions, CSH is very often diagnosed in elderly people (it occurs in 39% patients over the age of 65). However, some researchers have questioned these criteria and suggest that they should be modified. Krediet et al. [8] propose that the diagnosis of CSH should be based on the presence of asystole lasting at least 6 s in response to CSM and/or a fall in mean arterial pressure (MAP) to values below 60 mmHg for at least 6 s. In turn, Kerr et al. [7] suggested the occurrence of asystole lasting at least 7.3 s and/or a fall in systolic arterial pressure of more than 77 mmHg or both as diagnostic criteria. The incidence of CSH diagnosed using standard criteria and Krediet and Kerr criteria was 39%, 52% and 10%, respectively. On the basis of this study, it was demonstrated that CSH diagnosed using Kerr criteria was associated with increased all-cause mortality regardless of age and sex. The use of stricter Kerr criterion enables the distinguishing of a group of patients with the highest CSH-associated risk [19]. In 2013, Wieling et al. [9] suggested that all patients diagnosed with CSH should be treated as patients with mixed CSH and they presented new stricter set of criteria for the diagnosis of CSH occurrence.

Aetiology of CSS and CSH

The aetiology of CSS is unknown. The results of studies which aim was to explain CSS pathomechanism have failed to provide an unambiguous answer.

In 1799, Parry in his study demonstrated the existence of a significant relationship between carotid hypersensitivity and coronary disease and structural heart disease [1]. O'Mahony assumed that the ageing of our body and the progression of atherosclerotic lesions reduced carotid sinus wall compliance, resulting in the weakening of afferent pulse with the accompanying compensatory postsynaptic 'upregulation' of alpha-2 adrenoreceptors (central gain). Vigorous carotid sinus stimulation may result in an excessive efferent response causing a sudden pressure fall and/or asystole [20]. The hypothesis put forward by O'Mahony was not confirmed by Kenny et al. [21] or by Parry et al. [22].

The relationship between atherosclerotic lesions and CSH can be confirmed by a study conducted by Tsioufis et al. [23]. In their study, 118 participants underwent CSM before coronary angiography. CSH was found in 26.6% of patients and most of them had advanced multivessel coronary artery disease.

CSH is common in patients with neurodegenerative disorders and dementia. It was found in 40% of patients with Alzheimer's type dementia and in 50% of patients with dementia with Lewy bodies [17].

Carotid Artery Massage (CSM)

Over the years, many attempts have been made to find the optimal method of carotid sinus massage. Problem concerns the duration, the strength and the method of this massage. In 1932, Mandelstamm and Lifschitz suggested that the examined patient should be in a supine position with raised head [24]. They used the thumb to press for 10 to 20 s. Three researchers were necessary to perform their study: one of them was measuring a pressure, the second measured a pulse and the third pressed a carotid sinus. In 1933, Weiss and Baker noticed that it was easier to induce symptoms when patient was in upright position [4]. Novel techniques were searched for in the 1960s. In 1961, Lown and Levine proposed a method involving a gentle massage for 5 s [25]. In 1963, Franke published a technique involving 10–30 s stimulation which ended with the occurrence of asystole lasting 2–3 s [6]. In 1969, Thomas modified Franke's method. He started the test with a 20 s mild massage and ended it with a 15 s delicate longitudinal massage [14]. In the 1980s, longitudinal massage for less than 5 s with the use of pressure that did not hamper blood flow was considered to be a standard. At that time, there was no technical possibility to constantly measure heart rate or blood pressure during the massage. In 2004, the European Society of Cardiology issued recommendations regarding the diagnosis and the management of syncope according to which the massage can last from 5 to 10s [26].

Currently, carotid sinus massage can be performed both in a lying and standing position. Continuous monitoring of ECG and blood pressure is recommended. The massage is performed by compressing the right carotid artery for 5–10 s on the anterior margin of the sternocleidomastoid muscle at the level of the larynx. The CSM is presented in Fig. 3.1. If no positive massage result is observed, massage should be repeated on the opposite side after a break of 1–2 minutes. It is estimated that in 1/3 of patients, positive results of massage tests occur only during the

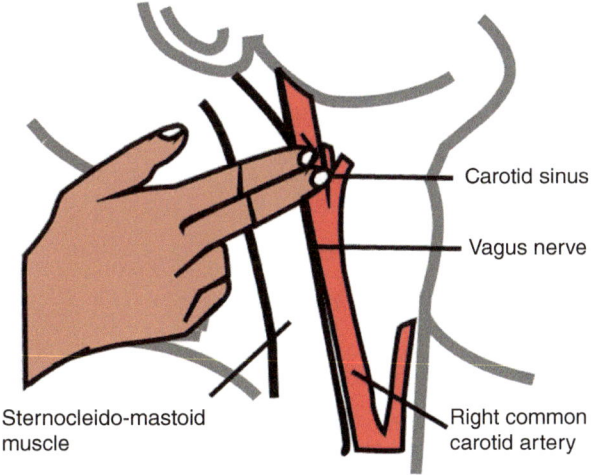

Fig. 3.1 Stimulation of carotid sinus triggers baroreceptor reflex and increased vagal tone, affecting SA and AV nodes

Carotid sinus

Vagus nerve

Sternocleido-mastoid muscle

Right common carotid artery

examination in a vertical position [11, 26–28]. A detailed description of the carotid sinus massage procedure can be found in the 2004 ESC Guidelines and in their update in 2018 [26, 29].

CSM is performed mainly for two reasons:

- In order to diagnose carotid sinus hypersensitivity in patients with syncope, dizziness, falls [30].
- In order to interrupt or to slow down supraventricular tachycardia (SVT) [25].

Contraindications

Carotid sinus massage is contraindicated in patients with: transient ischaemia or stroke during the last 3 months, audible murmur heard over a carotid artery, the presence of confirmed in ultrasound atherosclerotic plaques [31, 32].

Also a history of ventricular tachycardia or a previous myocardial infarction may be the contraindication to the test [32].

Complications

The most common complication following carotid sinus massage involve neurological complications. They occur relatively rarely. The results of 3 trials [32–34] in which a total of 7319 patients were examined indicate that neurological complications occurred in 21 (0.29%) people. The ESC guidelines of 2018 included data from the ESC guidelines from 2009 and the results of the subsequent study were added [35]. In the new population of 8720 patients, the number of patients with complications remained unchanged in comparison to previous data (21 cases). The percentage of patients with complications decreased to 0.24%.

CSS Treatment

The treatment of CSS depends on many factors, including the haemodynamic response to the carotid sinus massage and patient's clinical history. If there are obvious causative factors, such as vigorous rotation of the head or tight collars of a shirt, they should be eliminated in the first place [27].

Cardioinhibitory Type of CSS

According to ESC recommendations and on the basis of the results of available clinical trials, in case of cardioinhibitory form, cardiac pacing in class IIa is recommended [33, 36, 37]. Heart stimulation in CSS was for the first time used in 1970 by Voss in an 81-year-old female patient with recurrent syncope with asystole lasting

3.5 s during carotid sinus massage [38]. She was qualified for single-chamber pacemaker implantation (VVI). This treatment turned out to be effective in this patient.

Currently, two-chamber stimulation is preferred.

However, it has been observed that despite stimulation systems implantation, patients with CSS still suffer from recurrent syncope, however, they are less frequent in patients treated with electrotherapy in comparison with patients without an implanted pacemaker [39]. The scheme of management of cardioinhibitory CCS for patients over 40 years old is presented in Scheme 3.1. The positive tilt test response needs to be taken under consideration in order to counteract hypotensive susceptibility.

Evidence for the benefits of cardiac stimulation in patients with CSS is limited to several small control tests and retrospective studies. The frequency of syncope recurrence after pacemaker implantation ranges from 0% to 20%, while in patients without an implanted pacemaker, the recurrence rate is 20–60% [37]. In one of the registers of patient after pacemaker implantation, the recurrence rate was 7% in the first year, 16% in 3 years, and 20% in 5 years [33].

Brignole et al. [36] in their SUP2 study analysed the frequency of recurrent syncope in patients. Recurrent syncope rate in patients after pacemaker implantation was 9% in the first year, 18% in the second year and 20% in the third year in comparison to patients without stimulation in whom it was 21%, 33% and 43%, respectively. On the basis of this study, the class of the recommendation for implantation of a two-chamber pacemaker in patients with CSS was changed from class I to class IIa.

Vasodepressive Type of CSS

Patients with vasodepressive type of CSS are recommended to drink increased volume of fluid (more than 2 L/day) and to increase salt intake to 6 g/day, unless it is contraindicated (e.g. they do not suffer from hypertension). Moreover, the change of the method of antihypertensive treatment should also be considered [40].

The treatment of the vasodepressive type of CSS is difficult, and its results are generally unsatisfactory. Almquist et al. studied haemodynamic effects of various drug groups in patients with a pacemaker implanted due to a mixed form of CSS (vasodepressive and cardiodepressive). The results of their study demonstrated that atropine and propranolol did not prevent symptoms of vasodepression. The infusion of norepinephrine significantly reduced vasomotor response without a clear hypertensive response. A similar effect was obtained using ephedrine. However, adverse sympathomimetic effects disqualify these drugs from clinical use. The efficacy of isoproterenol and amphetamine was not confirmed [41].

In a non-randomized study [42] conducted on 11 patients with a vasodepressive form of CSS, patients received fludrocortisone in the dose of 100 μg and after 2 weeks they underwent repeated CSM. Significant decrease in vasodepressive reaction was observed. During the follow-up, patients also reported lower incidence of syncope symptoms.

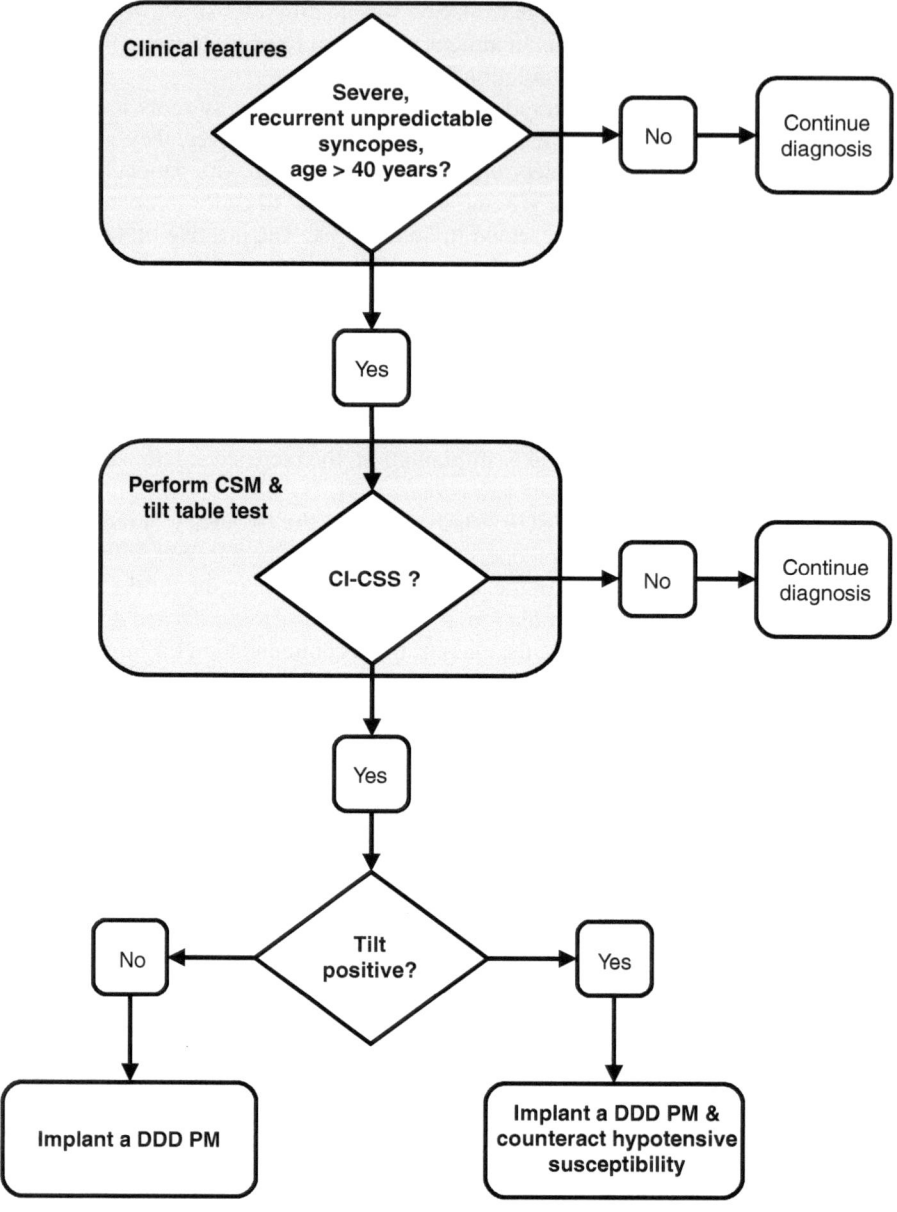

Scheme 3.1 Decision pathname for cardioinhibitory carotid sinus syndrome. CI-CSS, cardioin-hibitory carotid sinus syndrome; CSM, carotid sinus massage; DDD PM, dual chamber pacemaker

Grubb et al. [43] used in their study serotonin reuptake inhibitors (SSRIs). Their study comprised patients after pacemaker implantation due to cardioinhibitory form of CSS, who still suffered from syncope caused by vasodepressive component. Such treatment resulted in the relief of symptoms. However, due to the fact that only two patients participated in the study, it is not possible to formulate general conclusions regarding the treatment of patients suffering from CSS.

In another randomized, double-blind trial, patients with vasodepressive reaction were treated with midodrin [44]. Midodrin significantly reduced the symptoms but this treatment was associated with simultaneous occurrence of undesired pressure increase in ambulatory measurements. Therefore, midodrin therapy is of limited use in patients suffering from hypertension.

Beneficial effects of midodrin treatment were also observed in a study of Ward et al. [45] enrolling patients with hypotension and frequent syncope events.

In rare cases, the denervation of a carotid sinus with via surgery or irradiation has also been used. Despite the fact that this method has been known for over 60 years, it is not used [27, 31].

Prognosis

The prognosis of CSH and CSS is not entirely clear; recurrences of syncope occur both in persons with and without stimulation. Recurrent syncope may result in injuries and fractures.

Brignole et al. observed a group of 312 patients, 262 of whom were diagnosed with CSH. This group was compared with a group of 55 patients with unexplained syncope. There were no significant differences in the mortality rate in both groups. The mortality rate of patients in this study was similar to that of the general population [13].

Summary

Carotid sinus syndrome occurs mainly in elderly people. Carotid sinus massage is used to confirm carotid sinus hypersensitivity. The technique of carotid sinus massage has evolved along with the advancement of knowledge about carotid sinus syndrome and technical capacity to measure cardiac function and blood pressure in a continuous manner. At present, there is no common management scheme for the treatment of such patients. Depending on the patient's response, the cardioinhibitory and/or vasodepressive form can be distinguished. Patient's clinical history, age, gender, comorbidities and the results of available clinical trials should be considered before the choice of a treatment. There are no significant differences in mortality rates in patients with carotid sinus syndrome compared to mortality in the general population.

References

1. Parry CH. An inquiry into the symptoms and causes of the syncope anginosa commonly called angina pectoris. London: Bath; 1799.
2. Czermak J. Ueber mechanische Vagus-Reizung beim Menschen. Jenaische Zeitschrift fuer Medizin und Naturwissenschaft. 1866;2:384–6.
3. Roskam J. Un syndrome nouveau. Syncopes cardiaques graves et syncopes repetees par hyper-reflexivite sinocarotidienne. Presse Med. 1930;38:590–1.
4. Weiss S, Baker JP. The carotid sinus reflex in health and disease: its role in the causation of fainting and convulsions. Medicine Wien Arch f inn Med. 1933;12:297–354.
5. Nathanson MH. Hyperactive cardioinhibitory carotid sinus reflex. Arch Intern Med. 1946;77:491–503.
6. Franke H. On the hyperactive carotid sinus syndrome. Acta Neuroveg (Wien). 1963;25:187–203.
7. Kerr SR, Pearce MS, Brayne C, Davis RJ, Kenny RA. Carotid sinus hypersensitivity in asymptomatic older persons: implications for diagnosis of syncope and falls. Arch Intern Med. 2006;166:515–20.
8. Krediet CT, Parry SW, Jardine DL, Benditt DG, Brignole M, Wieling W. The history of diagnosing carotid sinus hypersensitivity: why are the current criteria too sensitive? Europace. 2011;13(1):14–22. https://doi.org/10.1093/europace/euq409. Epub 2010 Nov 17
9. Wieling W, Krediet CT, Solari D, de Lange FJ, van Dijk N, Thijs RD, van Dijk JG, Brignole M, Jardine DL. At the heart of the arterial baroreflex: a physiological basis for a new classification of carotid sinus hypersensitivity. J Intern Med. 2013;273(4):345–58. https://doi.org/10.1111/joim.12042.
10. The Task Force for the diagnosis and management of syncope of the European Society of Cardiology (ESC), 2018 ESC Guidelines for the diagnosis and management of syncope.
11. Gąsiorek PE, Banach M, Maciejewski M, Głąbiński A, Paduszyńska A, Rysz J, Bielecka-Dąbrowa A. Established and potential echocardiographic markers of embolism and their therapeutic implications in patients with ischemic stroke. Cardiol J. 2018; https://doi.org/10.5603/CJ.a2018.0046.
12. Sutton R. Carotid sinus syndrome: Progress in understanding and management. Glob Cardiol Sci Pract. 2014;2014(2):1–8. https://doi.org/10.5339/gcsp.2014.18. ECollection 2014
13. Brignole M, Oddone D, Cogorno S, Menozzi C, Gianfranchi L, Bertulla A. Long-term outcome in symptomatic carotid sinus hypersensitivity. Am Heart J. 1992;123(3):687–92.
14. Thomas JE. Hyperactive carotid sinus reflex and carotid sinus syncope. Mayo Clin Proc. 1969;44(2):127–39.
15. McIntosh SJ, Lawson J, Kenny RA. Clinical characteristics of vasodepressor, cardioinhibitory, and mixed carotid sinus syndrome in the elderly. Am J Med. 1993;95:203–8.
16. Amin V, Pavri BB. Carotid sinus syndrome. Cardiol Rev. 2015;23(3):130–4. https://doi.org/10.1097/CRD.0000000000000041.
17. Ballard C, Shaw F, McKeith L, Kenny R. High prevalence of neurovascular instability in neurodegenerative dementias. Neurology. 1998;51(6):1760–2.
18. Brignole M, Menozzi C. Carotid sinus syndrome: diagnosis, natural history and treatment. Eur J Card Pacing Electrophysiol. 1992;2:247–54.
19. McDonald C, Pearce MS, Newton JL, Kerr SR. Modified criteria for carotid sinus hypersensitivity are associated with increased mortality in a population-based study. Europace. 2016;18(7):1101–7. https://doi.org/10.1093/europace/euv219. Epub 2016 May 2
20. O'Mahony D. Pathophysiology of carotid sinus hypersensitivity in elderly patients. Lancet. 1995;346:950–2.
21. Kenny RA, Lyon CC, Ingram AM, et al. Enhanced vagal activity and normal arginine vasopressin response in carotid sinus syndrome: implications for a central abnormality in carotid sinus hypersensitivity. Cardiovasc Res. 1987;21:545–50.

22. Parry SW, Baptist M, Gilroy JJ, et al. Central alpha2 adrenoceptors and the pathogenesis of carotid sinus hypersensitivity. Heart. 2004;90:935–6.
23. Tsioufis CP, Kallikazaros IE, Toutouzas KP, et al. Exaggerated carotid sinus massage responses are related to severe coronary artery disease in patients being evaluated for chest pain. Clin Cardiol. 2002;25:161–6.
24. Mandelstamm M, Lifschitz S. Die Wirkung der Karotissinusreflexe auf den Blutdruck beim Menschen. Wien Arch F inn Med. 1932;22:397.
25. Lown B, Levine SA. The carotid sinus. Clinical value of its stimulation. Circulation. 1961;23:766–89.
26. Brignole M, Alboni P, Benditt DG, Bergfeldt L, Blanc JJ, Bloch Thomsen PE, van Dijk JG, Fitzpatrick A, Hohnloser S, Janousek J, Kapoor W, Kenny RA, Kulakowski P, Masotti G, Moya A, Raviele A, Sutton R, Theodorakis G, Ungar A, Wieling W, Task Force on Syncope, European Society of Cardiology. Guidelines on management (diagnosis and treatment) of syncope – update 2004. Europace. 2004;6:467–537.
27. Seifer C. Carotid sinus syndrome. Cardiol Clin. 2013;31(1):111–21. https://doi.org/10.1016/j.ccl.2012.10.002.
28. The Task Force for the Diagnosis and Management of Syncope of the European Society of Cardiology (ESC), Guidelines for the diagnosis and management of syncope (version 2009).
29. Brignole M, Moya A, de Lange FJ, Deharo JC, Elliott PM, Fanciulli A, Fedorowski A, Furlan R, Kenny RA, Martín A, Probst V, Reed MJ, Rice CP, Sutton R, Ungar A, van Dijk JG, ESC Scientific Document Group. Practical Instructions for the 2018 ESC Guidelines for the diagnosis and management of syncope. Eur Heart J. 2018;39(21):e43–80.
30. McIntosh S, da Costa D, Kenny RA. Benefits of an integrated approach to the investigation of dizziness, falls and syncope in elderly patients referred to a syncope clinic. Age Ageing. 1993;22:53–8.
31. Pasquier M, Clair M, Pruvot E, Hugli O, Carron PN. Carotid sinus massage. N Engl J Med. 2017;377(15):e21. https://doi.org/10.1056/NEJMvcm1313338.
32. Munro NC, McIntosh S, Lawson J, Morley CA, Sutton R, Kenny RA. The incidence of complications after carotid sinus massage in older patients with syncope. J Am Geriatr Soc. 1994;42:1248–51.
33. Puggioni E, Guiducci V, Brignole M, Menozzi C, Oddone D, Donateo P, Croci F, Solano A, Lolli G, Tomasi C, Bottoni N. Results and complications of the carotid sinus massage performed according to the 'methods of symptoms'. Am J Cardiol. 2002;89:599–60.
34. Davies AG, Kenny RA. Frequency of neurologic complications following carotid sinus massage. Am J Cardiol. 1998;81:1256–7.
35. Ungar A, Rivasi G, Rafanelli M, Toffanello G, Mussi C, Ceccofiglio A, McDonagh R, Drumm B, Marchionni N, Alboni P, Kenny RA. Safety and tolerability of Tilt Testing and Carotid Sinus Massage in the octogenarians. Age Ageing. 2016;45:242–8.
36. Brignole M, Arabia F, Ammirati F, Tomaino M, Quartieri F, Rafanelli M, Del Rosso A, Rita Vecchi M, Russo V, Gaggioli G, Syncope Unit Project 2 (SUP 2) investigators. Standardized algorithm for cardiac pacing in older patients affected by severe unpredictable reflex syncope: 3-year insights from the Syncope Unit Project 2 (SUP 2) study. Europace. 2016;18:1427–33.
37. Brignole M, Menozzi C. The natural history of carotid sinus syncope and the effect of cardiac pacing. Europace. 2011;13:462–4.
38. Voss DM, Magnin GE. Demand pacing and carotid sinus syncope. Am Heart J. 1970;79:544–7.
39. Claesson JE, Kristensson BE, Edvardsson N, et al. Less syncope and milder symptoms in patients treated with pacing for induced cardioinhibitory carotid sinus syndrome: a randomized study. Europace. 2007;9:932–6.
40. Solari D, Maggi R, Oddone D, Solano A, Croci F, Donateo P, Brignole M. Clinical context and outcome of carotid sinus syndrome diagnosed by means of the "method of symptoms". Europace. 2014;16(6):928–34.
41. Almquist A, Gornick C, Benson W. Carotid sinus hypersensitivity: evaluation of the vasodepressor component. Circulation. 1985;71(5):927–36.

42. DaCosta D, McIntosh S, Kenny RA. Benefits of fludrocortisone in the treatment of symptomatic vasodepressor carotid sinus syndrome. Br Heart J. 1993;69:308–10.
43. Grubb BP, Samoil D, Kosinski D, et al. The use of serotonin reuptake inhibitors for the treatment of recurrent syncope due to carotid sinus hypersensitivity unresponsive to dual chamber cardiac pacing. Pacing Clin Electrophysiol. 1994;17:1434–6.
44. Moore A, Watts M, Sheehy T, et al. Treatment of vasodepressor carotid sinus syndrome with midodrine: a randomized, controlled pilot study. J Am Geriatr Soc. 2005;53:114–8.
45. Ward CR, Gray JC, Gilroy JJ, Kenny RA. Midodrine: a role in the management of neurocardiogenic syncope. Heart. 1998;79(1):45–9.

Vasovagal Syncope

4

Kannayiram Alagiakrishnan

Introduction

Vasovagal syncope (VVS) is otherwise known as neurally mediated syncope. This was first described by Cotton and Lewis in 1918 [1]. This occurs due to a combination of vasodilatation and blood pressure drop (due to sympathetic withdrawal) and bradycardia (due to parasympathetic vagal disinhibition), and this vasodilatation and bradycardia occur simultaneously [2]. VVS can be inhibitory or vasodepressor or both. It is diagnosed using a head-up tilt test with continuous blood pressure and heart rate monitoring [3]. It is one of the main causes of presyncope and syncope in older adults [4].

Epidemiology

The incidence of VVS increases with aging [5]. In older adults, more than 50% of syncopal episodes are due to VVS. The lifetime incidence of an episode of VVS is more than 33% [6]. Rafanelli et al. showed in their study of 873 older adults that VVS was seen in 50.4% with neuro-mediated syncope subjects, and association with orthostatic hypotension was seen in 16% of these VVS patients [7]. EGSYS 2 (Evaluation of Guidelines in Syncope Study 2) study showed up to 66% had VVS [8], and GIS (Group for the Study of Syncope in the elderly) showed 62% in 65–75 years of age and 36.3% in more than 75 years [9, 10].

K. Alagiakrishnan (✉)
Division of Geriatric Medicine, University of Alberta, Edmonton, AB, Canada

© Springer Nature Switzerland AG 2020
K. Alagiakrishnan, M. Banach (eds.), *Hypotensive Syndromes in Geriatric Patients*, https://doi.org/10.1007/978-3-030-30332-7_4

Causes

Most of the time, the cause is unknown. It can be triggered by pain or emotional upset. A genetic link for the syndrome has been shown [11]. A Gly389 allele is more frequently present in VVS patients with a positive HUT test. The genetic basis is not very strong at this point [12]. Vasovagal syncope is commonly induced by triggers such as fear, pain, sight of blood, and instrumentation or precipitated by orthostatic or emotional stress and exposition to high environmental temperature.

Mechanisms

VVS is due to decrease in cardiac output as well as decrease in vascular tone. A combination of vasodilatation and blood pressure drop (due to sympathetic withdrawal) and bradycardia (due to parasympathetic vagal disinhibition) leads to VVS [2]. Mechanism of vasovagal syncope as a reflex arc is activated by afferent triggers which can result in presyncopal symptoms and the efferent effects causing vasodilation and bradycardia resulting in syncope. The inputs or afferent signals on parasympathetic system causing relative sinus bradycardia, sinus arrest as well as disappearance of sympathetic nervous system activation causing vasodilation and hypotension. In these processes, both parasympathetic activation and sympathetic inhibition are linked to VVS, but they do not always occur together and they can vary from one episode to another. Mechanisms leading to recovery from VVS are also unclear [13].

Vasovagal syncope is a reflex syncope resulting from a failure in autoregulation of blood pressure as well as cerebral perfusion pressure resulting in transient loss of consciousness. These reflex bradycardia and hypotension are similar to the response evoked by the Bezold–Jarisch reflex. VVS is characterised by periodic syncopal episodes with normal autonomic function between episodes. As mentioned earlier, vasodilatation and bradycardia occur simultaneously. The mechanism of the hypotension/bradycardia reflex responsible for VVS is not completely understood. Triggers such as emotional stress and pain stimulate the afferent limb of the reflex arc through the mechanoreceptors in the ventricles which stimulates the vagal afferents to the central nervous system. Along with it, central hypovolemia (from upright posture or dehydration) results in increased cardiac contractility in the setting of a relatively under-filled left ventricle. The efferent limb of the reflex arc results in increased parasympathetic activity with a decrease in heart rate and decreased sympathetic activity which decreases the vascular tone and a reduction in mean arterial blood pressure. When this falls below the cerebral autoregulation range, it could result in reduction in blood flow in the brain with loss of consciousness [14, 15].

Four phases of events are seen with VVS during active orthostatic stress like standing or passive orthostatic stress like tilt table testing: phase 1, early stabilisation; phase 2, circulatory instability (early presyncope); phase 3, terminal hypotension (late presyncope) and syncope; and phase 4, recovery. Fall in cardiac output is seen in older adults during phase 2 [16]. Decreased cardiac output is due to reduced baroreflex sensitivity (BRS) which can lead to VVS [17, 18].

Clinical Presentation

VVS can have typical or atypical presentation. In typical VVS, autonomic pro-dromes and loss of consciousness (LOC) are seen with triggers including orthostatic stress and tilt testing whereas with atypical VVS, episodes of LOC occur without any evident trigger and without prodromal symptoms and can be diagnosed only by tilt table testing. The prodromal symptoms include pallor, sweating, nausea, abdom-inal discomfort, feeling cold or feeling warm, palpitations, yawning, sighing, saliva-tion, dizziness, light headedness, and blurred vision. The precipitating triggers include prolonged standing (orthostatic stress), fear, severe pain, and sight of blood (emotional stress) [19, 20]. Atypical VVS is commonly seen in the elderly. LOC could start abruptly with a short prodrome leading to falls and injuries [21].

Two studies from Europe have investigated the spectrum of clinical features in patients with different phases of VVS. During the prodromal phase, blurred vision (27–68%), fatigue (23–68%), pallor (48–82%), sweating (32–66%), nausea (13–60%), palpitations (10–37%), feeling cold (12–29%), and feeling warm (6–18%), whereas prodromal symptoms were absent in 24–39% of subjects. In the syncopal phase, 13% had myoclonic jerks, incontinence up to 12% and minor trauma in up to 40%. During the recovery phase, symptoms were present in up to 76% of subjects [19, 22]. Few other studies pointed out that atypical presentation of VVS as a fall [23] as well as the syncope occurring in the lying position during the sleeping hours with the absence of any triggers [24, 25].

Evaluation/Diagnosis of VVS in Elderly

Persons with suspected VVS should undergo the following evaluation with different tests (Table 4.1). This will help to rule out other conditions [26].

1. Electrocardiogram (ECG): To look for evidence of underlying arrhythmogenic cardiac abnormalities, such as Wolff-Parkinson-White syndrome, prolonged QT syndrome, Brugada syndrome, or heart blocks.
2. Tilt table testing: This test measures the blood pressure and heart rate response to the change in position and also force of gravity. Tilt table testing is done in patients who have dizziness, falls, or syncope and helps to find out whether the abnormal blood pressure or heart rate contributes to these symptoms. This table

Table 4.1 Tests to be considered in the evaluation of VVS	
	1. ECG
	2. Blood pressure measurement with orthostatic stress/ active standing
	3. Holter monitoring, event monitoring, loop recorders
	4. Tilt table testing
	5. Carotid sinus massage
	6. Other tests

is a special table with the head end raised to 60–80 degrees with continuous monitoring of blood pressure and heart rate. During the tilt table testing, the sequence of hemodynamic events leading to vasovagal syncope can be divided into four phases as mentioned above. During phase 2, cardiac output falls in nearly all older adult patients [16]. Tilt testing, well tolerated even in the elderly, is useful in the differential diagnosis between vasovagal syncope and other forms of syncope, conditions leading to hypotension or autonomic dysfunction or falls. Tilt table testing has good specificity but low sensitivity (about 50%) and is not always reproducible (31–92%) [4, 27, 28].

3. Holter monitoring, event monitors, and loop recorders: VVS is difficult to capture. Holter monitoring is unlikely to be of benefit because of the short duration (24 hours) of monitoring. But it will help to exclude arrhythmias including bradyarrhythmias (such as sinus node dysfunction), atrioventricular conduction disorders, and tachyarrhythmias such as atrial fibrillation with rapid ventricular response and ventricular tachycardia as the cause of syncope [29]. Cardiac event portable recorders may be more useful as they allow for activation during symptoms and have to be used for days to weeks to record an event. Implantable loop recorders, which store 45 minutes of retrospective electrocardiographic data, may be more useful, and it can be activated by patients after each syncopal event [30].

4. Carotid sinus massage: Carotid sinus massage is a noninvasive diagnostic test used to detect carotid sinus hypersensitivity. It is done by gently massaging the carotid artery on one side of your neck for 5 seconds and the heart rhythm and blood pressure monitored during the massage. If carotid sinus is hypersensitive, with massage there will be a drop in blood pressure or slowed heart rate. Contraindications for doing this test include myocardial infarction (MI) or cerebrovascular accident (CVA) in the last 3 months, serious heart rhythm abnormalities like ventricular tachycardia or ventricular fibrillation [31].

5. Blood pressure measurement with orthostatic stress/active standing: This is most commonly used in patients with a high clinical probability of orthostatic hypotension (OH). Following a 5-minute period of rest in the supine position, BP measured in the supine position and an active stand of 3 minutes if tolerated [32].

6. Other tests: Hemoglobin, faecal occult blood test, electroencephalogram, computed tomography of the brain, echocardiogram, and electrophysiological studies.

Differential Diagnosis

Situational syncope must be excluded, as well as phobia syndromes or other organic causes. Because of the high prevalence of orthostatic hypotension (OH) and carotid sinus syndrome (CSS) in the elderly, these causes of syncope should be ruled out. OH should be ruled out by checking the blood pressure in lying and standing position and CSS by doing the carotid massage [33]. In elderly, presence of dyspnea and palpitations with syncope is suggestive of cardiac syncope, whereas with VVS one or more symptoms like nausea, sweating, blurred vision, and dizziness can occur before the episode [9]. Neurogenic syncope can occur with autonomic failure and epilepsy [34]. Polypharmacy-related syncope can occur in the elderly and is commonly seen with cardiovascular, neurological, and psychotropic medications [35] (Table 4.2).

Treatment/Management

Most of the time, vasovagal syncope is treated conservatively. The different therapeutic options include non-pharmacological, pharmacological, and cardiac pacing in selected patients [36, 37].

Non-pharmacological

Patients should be educated to recognise prodromal symptoms and instructed to place themselves in a supine position when they feel an event is coming. This can help to prevent syncope and reduces risk of falling and trauma. When known, patients

Table 4.2 Differential diagnosis of VVS

Condition	Prodromal symptoms	Precipitating factors	Diagnostic testing
VVS	Nausea, vomiting, abdominal pain, sweating, dizziness	Pain, sight of blood, emotional stress, fear, prolonged standing	Tilt table testing
Cardiac syncope	Dyspnea, palpitations	Severe aortic stenosis, severe heart failure, arrhythmias	Echocardiogram, Holter monitor
OH	Dizziness	Prolonged standing dehydration, medications	Checking BP in lying and standing
CSS	Dizziness	Mechanical manipulation of the carotid sinus in the neck by tight collars or shaving	Carotid sinus massage
Situational syncope	Phobia including feelings of dread or intense fear	Coughing, defaecation, micturition, post-exercise, panic attack	Medical and psychiatric assessment
Neurogenic syncope	Neurological symptoms	Autonomic failure, epilepsy	Autonomic function tests like Valsalva manoeuvre, deep breathing tests, cold pressor test
Polypharmacy related syncope	Dizziness, balance problems	Certain cardiovascular, psychotropic medications (neuroleptics, sedatives, antidepressants) and dopaminergic medications	Medication reconciliation

are instructed to avoid triggers. Like any other hypotensive syndromes, patients are also instructed to increase more water and fluid intake and physical countermeasures like leg-crossing and tensing of arm, abdominal, and buttock's muscles [38].

Pharmacological

If VVS is severe or not responding to conservative measures, medications like fludrocortisone, beta-blockers, and midodrine can be tried. The Prevention of Syncope Trial (POST) assessed the effectiveness of fludrocortisone and metoprolol and found these medications may be useful. The STAND trial did not show a significant improvement in symptoms with midodrine; however, a meta-analysis excluding the STAND trial found midodrine to be effective [39–43].

Pacemaker Therapy

VVS can be recurrent in some subjects especially with autonomic nervous system involvement, in spite of avoidance of triggers and using non-pharmacological approaches. The data at present do not show any effective pharmacological approach. In patients with severe bradycardias and asystole, pacemaker can be useful to prevent recurrent VVS. Especially in subjects with VVS with limited prodrome, without any triggers and documentation of severe bradycardia and asystole, as well as frequent recurrences with injuries, pacemaker therapy can be useful [44].

The North American Vasovagal Pacemaker Study (VPS) randomised patients with three or more episodes of syncope and a positive tilt table test (hypotension and relative bradycardia (<60/min)) to dual-chamber pacing versus no pacemaker. There was a 58% decreased risk of recurrent syncope in patients who were on the pacemaker therapy, 22% vs. 70%, $p = 0.00002$) [45]. In another multicentre randomised study, VASIS (Vasovagal Syncope International Study) subjects with three or more syncopal episodes compared standard therapy with pacing over 2 years. There was 56% reduction in syncope with pacemaker (61% vs. 5%, $p = 0.0006$) [46]. In refractory or disabling cases of VVS with cardioinhibitory response or prolonged asystole, cardiac pacing especially closed loop stimulation (CLS) is a therapeutic option. Several RCT studies showed its usefulness. In a randomised, single-blind, crossover study in refractory vasovagal syncope, the effect of dual-chamber CLS was assessed in the prevention of syncope recurrence up to 36 months [47]. The ISSUE-3 study also found significant benefit ($p < 0.039$) in prevention of syncope recurrence in older patients as well as other studies with implantable rhythm devices [30, 48–52].

VVS and Quality of Life (QoL)

VVS is associated with reduced quality of life in older subjects [53–56]. In subjects with recurrent VVS, especially highly symptomatic as well as related to psychiatric disorders are associated with a reduced health- related quality of life

(HRQoL) [57, 58]. In another study over a period of 6 months, the common QoL questionnaire, the Short Form 36 questionnaire (SF-36) which covers seven dimensions of QoL, was prospectively administrated to all consecutive VVS patients. Those patients who had recurrent VVS had a worse QoL [59]. A study showed that in patients with frequent recurrences of VVS, non-pharmacological treatment had a beneficial effect on both syncopal recurrence and QoL [60].

Driving Issues Related to Syncope

Healthcare providers should warn patients about risk with driving and discuss about public safety. Most people with rare episodes of vasovagal syncope can drive safely. Legal restrictions on the ability to drive with recurrent syncope vary significantly with different jurisdictions. For personal vehicle, it may be for 3 months, and for commercial vehicles, it may be 6 months of symptom-free period [61, 62].

Prevention of VVS

The best way to prevent vasovagal response is to avoid common triggers. If not possible, these are some of the steps patient can take to manage those triggers and prevent a syncopal episode: (1) avoid hot, crowded, and stuffy areas; (2) drink plenty of fluids and increase salt intake if possible; (3) avoid standing for a long time, and if necessary to stand for a long time, keep tensing your leg muscles to keep the leg circulation moving; (4) avoid syncopal or fainting spells, and cross the legs and not the fingers; and (5) during blood withdrawal, sit or lie down.

Conclusions

VVS is the most common type of reflex syncope. There has been significant progress in recent years regarding the understanding and management of VVS. There are two main types: vasodepressor (associated with hypotension) and cardioinhibitory type (associated with bradycardia). Atypical presentation is common in the elderly. In some patients, it is self-limited, while in others, it can cause recurrent episodes. Management include patient education, non-pharmacological conservative management, and medical management including pacing therapy for cardioinhibitory type.

References

1. Cotton TF, Lewis T. Observations upon fainting attacks due to inhibitory cardiac impulses. Heart. 1918;7:23–4.
2. Morillo CA, Eckberg DL, Ellenbogen KA, et al. Vagal and sympathetic mechanisms in patients with orthostatic vasovagal syncope. Circulation. 1997;96:2509–13.
3. Alboni P, Brignole M, degli Uberti EC. Is vasovagal syncope a disease? Europace. 2007;9:83–7.

4. Parry SW, Kenny RA. The role of tilt table testing in neurocardiovascular instability in older adults. Eur Heart J. 2001;22(5):370–2.
5. Colman N, Nahm K, Ganzeboom KS, et al. Epidemiology of reflex syncope. Clin Auton Res. 2004;14:9–17.
6. Hogan TM, Constantine ST, Crain AD. Evaluation of syncope in older adults. Emerg Med Clin North Am. 2016;34(3):601–27.
7. Rafanelli M, Morrione A, Landi A, et al. Neuroautonomic evaluation of patients with unexplained syncope: incidence of complex neurally mediated diagnoses in the elderly. Clin Interv Aging. 2014;9:333–8.
8. Brignole M, Ungar A, Bartoletti A, et al. Standardized-care pathway vs usual management of syncope patients presenting as emergencies at general hospitals. Europace. 2006;8:644–50.
9. Galizia G, Abete P, Mussi C, et al. Role of early symptoms in assessment of syncope in elderly people: results from the Italian group for the study of syncope in the elderly. J Am Geriatr Soc. 2009;57:18–23.
10. Del Rosso A, Ungar A, Bartoli P, et al. Usefulness and safety of shortened head-up tilt testing potentiated with sublingual glyceryl trinitrate in older patients with recurrent unexplained syncope. J Am Geriatr Soc. 2002;50:1324–8.
11. Lelonek M. Genetics in neurocardiogenic syncope. Przegl Lek. 2006;63(12):1310–2.
12. Olde Nordkamp LR, Wieling W, Zwinderman AH, et al. Genetic aspects of vasovagal syncope: a systematic review of current evidence. Europace. 2009;11(4):414–20.
13. Adkisson WO, Benditt DG. Pathophysiology of reflex syncope: a review. J Cardiovasc Electrophysiol. 2017;28(9):1088–97.
14. Wallin BG, Sundlöf G. Sympathetic outflow to muscle during vasovagal syncope. J Auton Nerv Syst. 1982;6:287–91.
15. Jardine DL, Melton IC, Crozier JG, et al. Decrease in cardiac output and muscle sympathetic activity occurs during vasovagal syncope. Am J Physiol Heart Circ Physiol. 2002;282:H1804–9.
16. Jardine DL, Wieling W, Brignole M, et al. Pathophysiology of the vasovagal response. Heart Rhythm. 2018;15(6):921–9.
17. Mitro P, Simurda M, Evin L, et al. Reduced baroreflex sensitivity in patients with vasovagal syncope. Bratisl Lek Listy. 2015;116(10):582–6.
18. Iacoviello M, Forleo C. Guida pet al.Independent role of reduced arterial baroreflex sensitivity during head-up tilt testing in predicting vasovagal syncope recurrence. Europace. 2010;12(8):1149.
19. Alboni P, Brignole M, Menozzi C, et al. Clinical spectrum of neurally mediated reflex syncope. Europace. 2004;6:55–62.
20. Accurso V, Winnicki M, Shamsuzzmam ASM, et al. Predisposition to vasovagal syncope in subjects with blood/injury phobia. Circulation. 2001;104:903–7.
21. Del Rosso A, Alboni P, Brignole M, et al. Relation of clinical presentation of syncope tothe age of patients. Am J Cardiol. 2006;96:1431–5.
22. Graham LA, Kenny RA. Clinical characteristics of patients with vasovagal reactions presenting as unexplained syncope. Europace. 2001;3:141–6.
23. Rafanelli M, Ruffolo E, Chisciotti VM, et al. Clinical aspects and diagnostic relevance of neuroanatomic evaluation in patients with unexplained falls. Aging Clin Exp Res. 2014;26:33–7.
24. Krediet CTP, Jardine DL, Cortelli P, et al. Vasovagal syncope interrupting sleep? Heart. 2004;90:e25.
25. Alboni P. The different clinical presentations of vasovagal syncope. Heart. 2015;101:674–8.
26. Parry SW, Tan MP. An approach to the evaluation and management of syncope in adults. BMJ. 2010;340:c880.
27. Benditt DG, Ferguson DW, Grubb DW, et al. Tilt table testing for assessing syncope. J Am Coll Cardiol. 1996;28:263–75.
28. Forleo C, Guida P, Iacoviello M, et al. Head-up tilt testing for diagnosing vasovagal syncope: a meta-analysis. Int J Cardiol. 2013;169:e49–50.
29. Seipel L. The clinical value of Holter ECG recording. Internist. 2004;45:1035–41.
30. Brignole M, Sutton R, Menozzi C, et al. Early application of an implantable loop recorder allows effective specific therapy in patients with recurrent suspected neurally mediated syncope. Eur Heart J. 2006;27:1085–92.

31. Brignole M, Moya A, de Lange FJ, et al. ESC Scientific Document Group. Practical instructions for the 2018 ESC guidelines for the diagnosis and management of syncope. Eur Heart J. 2018;39(21):e43–80.

32. Consensus statement on the definition of orthostatic hypotension, pure autonomic failure, and multiple system atrophy. The Consensus Committee of the American Autonomic Society and the American Academy of Neurology. Neurology. 1996;46(5):1470.

33. Nwazue VC, Raj SR. Confounders of vasovagal syncope: orthostatic hypotension. Cardiol Clin. 2013;31:89.

34. Dantas FG, Cavalcanti AP, Rodrigues Maciel BD, et al. The role of EEG in patients with syncope. J Clin Neurophysiol. 2012;29:55–7.

35. Ruwald MH, Hansen ML, Lamberts M, et al. Comparison of incidence, predictors and the impact of co- morbidity and polypharmacy on the risk of recurrent syncope in patients <85 versus ≥85 years of age. Am J Cardiol. 2013;112:1610–5.

36. Parry SW, Kenny RA. The management of vasovagal syncope. Q J Med. 1999;92:697–705.

37. Kenny RA, McNicholas T. The management of vasovagal syncope. QJM Int J Med. 2016;109(12):767–73.

38. van Dijk N, Quartieri F, Blanc JJ, et al. Effectiveness of physical counter pressure maneuvers in preventing vasovagal syncope: the Physical Counter pressure Manoeuvres Trial (PC-Trial). J Am Coll Cardiol. 2006;48:1652–7.

39. Sheldon R, Connolly S, Rose S, et al. Prevention of Syncope Trial (POST): a randomized, placebo-controlled study of metoprolol in the prevention of vasovagal syncope. Circulation. 2006;113:1164–70.

40. Sheldon R, Raj SR, Rose MS, et al. POST 2 Investigators. Fludrocortisone for the prevention of vasovagal syncope: a randomized, placebo-controlled trial. J Am Coll Cardiol. 2016;68(1):1–9.

41. Romme JJ, van Dijk N, Go-Schon IK, et al. Effectiveness of midodrine treatment in patients with recurrent vasovagal syncope not responding to non-pharmacological treatment (STAND-trial). Europace. 2011;13:1639–47.

42. Vyas A, Swaminathan PD, Zimmerman MB, Olshansky B. Are treatments for vasovagal syncope effective? A meta-analysis. Int J Cardiol. 2013;167:1906–11.

43. Schleifer JW, Shen WK. Vasovagal syncope: an update on the latest pharmacological therapies. Expert Opin Pharmacother. 2015;16:501–13.

44. Shen WK, Sheldon RS, Benditt DG, et al. 2017 ACC/AHA/HRS guideline for the evaluation and management of patients with syncope. Circulation. 2017;136:e25–59.

45. Connolly SJ, Sheldon R, Roberts RS, Gent M. The North American Vasovagal Pacemaker Study (VPS 1). A randomized trial of permanent cardiac pacing for the prevention of vasovagal syncope. J Am Coll Cardiol. 1999;33:16–20.

46. Sutton R, Brignole M, Menozzi C, et al. Dual-chamber pacing in the treatment of neurally mediated tilt-positive cardioinhibitory syncope: pacemaker versus no therapy. Circulation. 2000;102:294–9.

47. Russo V, Rago A, Papa AA, et al. The effect of dual-chamber closed-loop stimulation on syncope recurrence in healthy patients with tilt-induced vasovagal cardioinhibitory syncope. Heart. 2013;99:1609–13.

48. Connolly SJ, Sheldon R, Thorpe KE, et al. Pacemaker therapy for prevention of syncope in patients with recurrent severe vasovagal syncope: second vasovagal pacemaker study (VPS 11): a randomized trial. J Am Med Assoc. 2003;289(17):2224–9.

49. Raviele A, Giada F, Menozzi C, et al. A randomized, double-blind, placebo-controlled study of permanent cardiac pacing for the treatment of recurrent tilt-induced vasovagal syncope. The vasovagal syncope and pacing trial (SYNPACE). Eur Heart J. 2004;25(19):1741–8.

50. Brignole M, Menozzi C, Moya A, et al. Pacemaker therapy in patients with neurally mediated syncope and documented asystole: third international study on syncope of uncertain etiology (ISSUE-3): a randomized trial. Circulation. 2012;125(21):2566–71.

51. Palmisano P, Zaccaria M, Luzzi G, et al. Closed-loop cardiac pacing vs. conventional dual-chamber pacing with specialized sensing and pacing algorithms for syncope prevention in patients with refractory vasovagal syncope: results of a long-term follow-up. Europace. 2012;14(7):1038–43.

52. Solbiati M, Sheldon RS. Implantable rhythm devices in the management of vasovagal syncope. Auton Neurosci. 2014;184:33–9.
53. Baron-Esquivias G, Gomez S, Aguilera A, et al. Short-term evolution of vasovagal syncope: influence on the quality of life. Int J Cardiol. 2005;102:315–9.
54. Giada F, Silvestri I, Rossillo A, et al. Psychiatric profile, quality of life and risk of syncopal recurrence in patients with tilt-induced vasovagal syncope. Europace. 2005;7:465–71.
55. Gracie J, Newton J, Norton M, et al. The role of psychological factors in response to treatment in neurocardiogenic(vasovagal) syncope. Europace. 2006;8:636–43.
56. Shaffer C, Jackson L, Jarecki S. Characteristics, perceived stressors, and coping strategies of patients who experience neurally mediatedsyncope. Heart Lung. 2001;30:244–9.
57. Rose MS, Koshman ML, Spreng S, Sheldon R. The relationship between health-related quality of life and frequency of spells in patients with syncope. J Clin Epidemiol. 2000;53:1209–16.
58. Giada F, Silvestri I, Rosillo A, et al. Psychiatric profile, quality of life and risk of syncopal recurrence in patients with tilt-induced vasovagal syncope. Eur Secur. 2005;7(5):465–71.
59. Baron- Esquivias G, Gomez S, Aguilera A, et al. Short-term evolution of vasovagal syncope: influence on the quality of life. Int J Cardiol. 2005;102(2):315–9.
60. Romme JJ, Reitsma JB, Go- Schon IK, et al. Prospective evaluation of non- pharmacological treatment in vasovagal syncope. Europace. 2010;12(4):567–73.
61. Li H, Weitcel M, Easley A. Potential risk of vasovagal syncope for motor vehicle driving. Am J Cardiol. 2000;85:184–6.
62. Guzman J, Morillo CA. Syncope and driving. Cardiol Clin. 2015;33:465–71.

Post-exercise Hypotension in the Elderly

Agata Bielecka-Dabrowa, Marcin Adam Bartłomiejczyk, Marek Maciejewski, and Maciej Banach

Introduction

Hypertension is the most common, costly, and preventable cardiovascular disease (CVD) risk factor, affecting 1.4 billion (31%) adults in the world [1, 2]. Keeping this growing and costly public health crisis in check with the adoption and maintenance of lifestyle interventions such as habitual physical activity is a national and global priority [1, 3]. Engaging in regular exercise is also recommended as a means to reduce resting blood pressure (BP) values.

Exercise is considered a form of ischemic preconditioning, and individuals who exercise regularly would have a smaller infarct size and overall improved left ventricular systolic function when encountering a clinical ischemic event, such as an acute myocardial infarction (MI) [4]. The beneficial effects of exercise preconditioning or post-exercise hypotension on endothelial function and the myocardium may be mediated via increased blood flow, enhanced nitric oxide production and bioavailability, changes in neurohormone release, improvements in oxidant/antioxidant balance, and optimization of energy and adenosine triphosphate (ATP)

A. Bielecka-Dabrowa (✉) · M. Banach
Department of Hypertension, Chair of Nephrology and Hypertension, Medical University of Lodz, Lodz, Poland

Department of Cardiology and Congenital Diseases of Adults, Polish Mother's Memorial Hospital Research Institute (PMMHRI), Lodz, Poland
e-mail: agata.bielecka-dabrowa@iczmp.edu.pl; maciej.banach@umed.lodz.pl

M. A. Bartłomiejczyk
Department of Hypertension, Medical University of Lodz, Lodz, Poland

M. Maciejewski
Department of Cardiology and Congenital Diseases of Adults, Polish Mother's Memorial Hospital Research Institute (PMMHRI), Lodz, Poland

© Springer Nature Switzerland AG 2020
K. Alagiakrishnan, M. Banach (eds.), *Hypotensive Syndromes in Geriatric Patients*, https://doi.org/10.1007/978-3-030-30332-7_5

metabolism. It is likely that many, or all, of these factors contribute to the cardiovascular health benefits from exercise [4].

A single bout of exercise can lead to a post-exercise decrease in BP, a phenomenon known as post-exercise hypotension (PEH) [5, 6]. The effect of acute hypotension has an important clinical relevance after both aerobic and resistance exercises, because it can last up to 24–48 hours post-exercise.

Aerobic exercise training lowers blood pressure (BP) from 5 to 7 mmHg among adults with hypertension [7, 8]. Therefore, professional organizations throughout the world recommend regular participation in aerobic exercise for the prevention, treatment, and control of hypertension [7].

The chronic BP reductions resulting from aerobic exercise training are largely due to PEH [9–11], although the mechanisms that mediate the acute and chronic exercise BP effects may differ [12–14]. It is worth pointing out that reductions of around 5 mmHg in BP reduce the risk of stroke mortality by 14% and coronary heart disease by 9% [15].

Studies report that PEH is directly linked to baseline BP: the higher the values, the greater the magnitude of reduced BP [12, 16]. Interestingly, several studies have demonstrated that longer exercise bouts lead to a greater and longer PEH [12, 16].

In the meta-analysis of Carpio-Rivera et al. [17] based on 65 studies, the reduction in BP was significant regardless of the participant's initial BP level, gender, physical activity level, antihypertensive drug intake, type of BP measurement, time of day in which the BP was measured, type of exercise performed, and exercise training program (p < 0.05 for all). However, the hypotensive effect was greater when the exercise was performed as a preventive strategy in those physically active and without antihypertensive medication.

Despite the documented antihypertensive benefits of acute (PEH) and chronic (training) aerobic exercise, there is significant interindividual variability in the BP response to exercise. Investigators from the HEalth, RIsk Factors, Exercise TrAining and GEnetics, or HERITAGE, Family Study involving over 700 white and black subjects have established the BP response to acute and chronic aerobic exercise is heritable with evidence of a shared genetic influence [14, 18–25].

The Postulated Mechanisms of PEH

The mechanism of PEH and its relationship with cardiovascular protection is not fully understood. The postulated mechanisms for post-exercise blood pressure reduction are a decrease in peripheral vascular resistance, reduction in cardiac output, release of vasodilatory substances [26–30], increase in histamine activity [31], reduction in sympathetic nerve activity [32], and possible improvement of the antioxidant system [33].

Dudzinska and colleagues [34] have shown in healthy subjects that exercise increased production of ATP in the red blood cells (RBC). The effect was specific mainly to adenine nucleotide metabolism and did not affect metabolism of guanine and pyridine nucleotides in the RBC.

The exercise and the post-exercise effect is mediated by increased metabolism and production of ATP in RBCs and other cell types, which would preserve, either directly or indirectly, intracellular ATP concentration when encountering an insult induced by oxidative stress and/or cardiovascular injury. It is probable that one of the mechanisms of post-exercise hypotension is via an increase in ATP metabolism in the RBC, which, if proven correct, will provide a surrogate biomarker for developing novel strategy for cardiovascular prevention and protection [34].

A single bout of aerobic exercise produces a post-exercise hypotension associated with a sustained post-exercise vasodilation of the previously exercised muscle [35]. During the exercise recovery period, the combination of centrally mediated decreases in sympathetic nerve activity with a reduced signal transduction from sympathetic nerve activation into vasoconstriction, as well as local vasodilator mechanisms, contributes to the fall in arterial blood pressure seen after exercise. Important findings from recent studies include the recognition that skeletal muscle afferents may play a primary role in post-exercise resetting of the baroreflex via discrete receptor changes within the nucleus tractus solitarii and that sustained post-exercise vasodilation of the previously active skeletal muscle is primarily the result of histamine H1 and H2 receptor activation (Fig. 5.1).

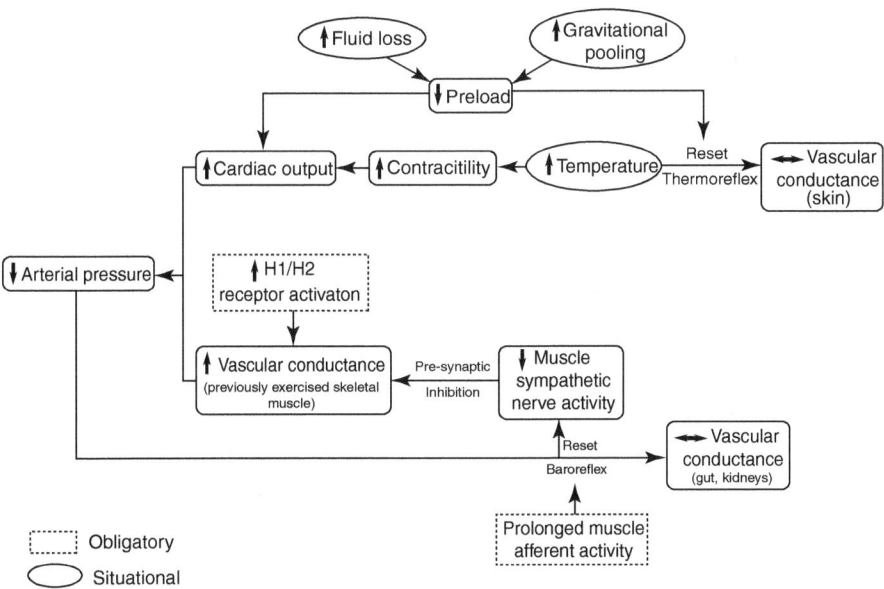

Fig. 5.1 Integrated hemodynamic responses following exercise. Post-exercises hypotension outcomes from the integration of diversity of situation and obligatory components. The obligatory components contain elements such as: (1) persistent dilatation of histaminergic blood vessels of the previously exercised skeletal muscle vascular beds; (2) presynaptic inhibition of noradrenaline release from sympathetic nerves to the exercised muscle; and resetting of (3) thermoreflexes and (4) baroreflex. These changes manifest themselves as an increase in the vascular conduction of the previously performed muscle, inhibition of sympathetic activity of narrowing blood vessels nerve activity to muscle vascular beads, and no or little change in cutaneous vascular conductance in spite of higher core temperatures. Situational components contain the effect of significant or non-significant fluid loss, gravitational pooling of blood, and hyperthermia are present. These ingredients may have a big impact on the degree to which cardiac output is elevated

Regarding the possible underlying mechanisms, Ray and Carrasco [36] reported that isometric handgrip (IHD) training may reduce BP levels by improving endothelial function; thus, isometric exercise would increase the bioavailability of nitric oxide (NO^-) derived from the endothelium, which has a vasodilator action. In addition, Clifford and Hellsten [37] also suggested that lactate could contribute to local vasodilation via NO synthase, thus allowing BP reduction after exercise. Nevertheless, the mechanisms responsible for the reduction of BP at rest acutely after exercise have not been fully clarified.

Different Types of Exercises and PEH

Besides aerobic exercising, resistance training is also recommended for hypertensive individuals as a form of increasing muscle strength [12]. However, although showing promising results, research on the occurrence of PEH in hypertensive individuals engaged in this type of exercise is scarce [38–42]. Moreover, there are differences in experimental protocols, such as weight load, number of repetitions, and quantity of exercises. Although there are several studies on the subject, an analysis is still lacking on a state-of-art approach considering different types of exercises.

In a few previous studies carried out in elderly individuals with hypertension, significant decreases in systolic and diastolic blood pressure were observed after 45 minutes of aerobic exercise performed at low to moderate intensities (i.e., 50% VO_2 max) [43] and high intensities (i.e., above 70% VO_2 max) [44]. Additionally, different volumes of resistance exercise (e.g., 1 and 3 sets) reduced blood pressure during 90 min after exercise with more pronounced effects observed in the exercise session with higher volume [45].

Apparently, aerobic exercises promote a greater and longer reduction in BP levels than resistance exercises. However, further studies applying resistance exercise in hypertensive individuals are necessary [26]. There is not one prescription model for weight training exercise that can promote greater reductions in the blood pressure values of hypertensive individuals. However, considering the individuals' safety, the exercise intensity should be around 50% of repetition maximum, with a minimum of one-minute intervals (between sets and exercises), using especially the great muscle groups. Moreover, long series of exercises that leads to exhaustion should be avoided, as they can induce greater BP increases [26].

In most studies, the prescription of aerobic activities ranged from 50% to 60% of the VO_2 max. performed continuously during 30 to 45 minutes. It is significant that there are still findings that conflict relative to the best intensity and duration of this modality of exercise.

Recent studies attempted to determine whether resistance exercise alone could produce the same hypotensive effect as aerobic exercise [46–48].

Melo et al. [38] revealed that in hypertensive women receiving captopril, a single bout of low-intensity resistance exercise reduced blood pressure. This reduction persists for 10 h, during the awake period, while patients were engaged in their daily living activities and it was greater in patients with higher ambulatory blood pressure. In the study of Brito et al. [49], high-intensity resistance exercise was effective in promoting PEH, this phenomenon being accompanied by a reduction in forearm vascular resistance within the first minute of recovery in the hypertensive elderly. The results of Freitas et al. [50] suggest that resistance exercise of higher intensity promoted greater post-exercise hypotension accompanied by greater increases in forearm blood flow, vasodilator response, heart rate, and cardiac sympathovagal balance. Also, the same authors conclude that a single resistance exercise session with three series was able to promote higher PEH in hypertensive women than exercise with one set, and this phenomenon was accompanied by increased forearm blood flow and increased cardiac autonomic activity [51].

The type of exercise is also important. An acute bout of aquatic treadmill (ATM) induced a more favorable endothelial response and greater post-exercise hypotensive response than land treadmill (LTM) [52]. These changes were associated with increased atrial natriuretic peptide (ANP) levels following ATM. Despite the potential benefits of dynamic resistance training, many of the elderly in long-term care institutions are considered to be physically less active among the older population. In addition, the changes that occur with aging can lead to mobility problems in the elderly and have a higher complexity of executing movements using dynamic resistance exercise [53]. At last, the use of robust and costly equipment makes it difficult to structure gyms in long-term care institutions, clinics, and hospitals that care for the elderly [54]. On the other hand, the use of portable dynamometers (e.g., handgrip), with low cost in relation to gym equipment, are easy to understand and execute, have quick adherence, and can collaborate as an adjuvant in the control, treatment, and prevention of hypertension [55–58]. Evidence suggests that IHG training (chronic) can be applied as an important adjuvant tool in hypertension. The study of Souza et al. [59] found that a single session of IHG of moderate-intensity with greater overload of work reduces systolic blood pressure (SBP) values from −14.4 to −18.7 mmHg between 10 and 60 min post-exercise in the hypertensive elderly people. One of the major concerns of resistance exercise in hypertensive patients is the question of cardiovascular safety and elevated BP responses during exercise [12, 16]. This study observed that 1 min after the IHG exercise session, all cardiovascular parameters returned to the baseline values. These results agree with other studies examining IHG exercise [60]. Thus, this type of IHG exercise, with mild to moderate intensity, with short contraction times, appears to be safe for this population.

In recent years, it has been recognized that concurrent training (i.e., a combination of resistance and aerobic exercises) is the most effective strategy to improve both neuromuscular and cardiovascular outcomes in elderly individuals [61].

Ferrari R et al. [62] evaluated BP responses after concurrent resistance and aerobic exercises in elderly men with essential hypertension. They found that the concurrent exercise reduced BP in the first hour after the exercise session and that the reduction was similar to the aerobic exercise alone. However, sustained reductions in diastolic blood pressure observed in the aerobic exercise session were not replicated after the concurrent exercise. These results suggest that an acute bout of concurrent exercise would produce PEH similar to aerobic exercise, but such effect may not last as long as aerobic exercise in elderly patients with essential hypertension.

Their finding highlights the use of aerobic exercise as gold standard exercise to reduce BP.

In the meta-analysis by Carpio-Rivera et al. [17], both aerobic and resistance exercises alone were able to induce a hypotensive effect. The authors found jogging to be the exercise modality that elicits the greater magnitude of systolic BP and diastolic BP changes. Other findings were that walking does not reduce the diastolic BP; that the longer the duration of the exercise session, the greater the systolic BP reduction; and that incremental exercise protocols produce the highest reductions in systolic BP. These findings seem to agree with a previous report [63] that associated the PEH with the total exercise workload and not with the intensity at which the exercise was performed.

Post meta-analytical studies assessing resistance training programs are needed, since reductions in diastolic BP were found with a greater number of resistance exercises, although these exercises also led to a minor decrease in systolic BP.

The Factors Influencing PEH

Physically active individuals achieved higher BP decreases after the exercise session. This was observed even though the PEH occurred independently from the level of physical activity of the participants. This seems to support the theory proposed by some authors [64] who observed that some physiological mechanisms that chronically reduce BP also play a role in the onset of PEH. For example, exercise training has been shown to cause a systemic adaptation of the arterial wall in healthy individuals [65], which might translate to better arterial vessel compliance that may facilitate the decrease in peripheral resistance following an exercise session.

The lower body mass index (BMI) is associated with a greater reduction in systolic BP what is in line with evidence showing that adipose tissue accumulation, especially in the abdominal area, is linked to several mechanisms leading to hypertension, including sympathetic overactivity, endothelial dysfunction, arterial stiffness, and inflammation [64, 66, 67]. Therefore, maintaining a normal BMI could lead in many cases to a greater hypotensive effect following an exercise session [68].

In the meta-analysis of Cardio-Rivera et al. [17], an inverse association between age and PEH was observed. Increasing age decreases the magnitude of PEH. As a person ages, there is an increase in arterial stiffness that results from progressive destruction of the elastic fibers, a decrease in capillary density, and an increase in arteriolar wall thickness. These structural and functional changes, in turn, increase vascular resistance and limit the response to vasodilator agents released during exercise [69]. Similarly, if the VO_2 max is greatest when the person is young and active, then the relationship between a higher VO_2 max and a greater decrease in systolic BP could also be explained by the aforementioned physiological mechanisms.

Dietary plans, such as the Dietary Approaches to Stop Hypertension (DASH) diet proposed by the National Heart, Lung, and Blood Institute of the United States, and several specific foods are known to promote BP reduction [70]. Among these foods, purple grapes and derivatives have shown a high capacity to reduce BP in animal models and in a human hypertension model [71–75]; this effect is attributed to their rich polyphenol composition, with the main component being flavonoids, which have vasodilator [76] and antioxidant [77] properties, allowing these foods to exert effects similar to those of moderate and regular physical exercise.

The study of Neto et al. [78] showed that a 28-day grape juice supplementation protocol promotes a reduction in the BP at rest and improves PEH but only in individuals with hypertension with an systolic BP between 120 and 140 mmHg and a diastolic BP between 80 and 90 mmHg. Individuals with better controlled hypertension with a pressure lower than 120/80 mmHg were not responsive to grape juice in terms of BP at rest and did not show PEH prior to nutritional intervention but began to present a post-exercise BP reduction after 28 days of supplementation with whole red grape juice.

Considering that there are individuals with hypertension resistant to the pressure reduction promoted by exercise [79–83], even when the subjects begin sessions with high BP, the study of Neto et al. [78] suggests that the possibility that grape juice or other nutritional agents can restore the post-exercise hypotensive capacity of these people should be investigated.

A meta-regression of 187 studies to assess the overall prevalence of anabolic-androgenic steroids (AAS) concluded that nonmedical AAS use is a serious, widespread public health problem that has a high prevalence in different populations and demonstrated an incapability of AAS users to obtain a reduction in blood pressure after an aerobic exercise session [84].

Coffee is a widely consumed beverage on a daily basis, second only to water in the United States [85]. However, this exercise-induced blood pressure response is also influenced by caffeine ingestion, as demonstrated by studies [86] in which the intravenous or oral administration of 4 mg of caffeine per kilogram of body weight (equivalent to three doses of coffee) blunted the PEH. The studies confirmed that the consumption of coffee or caffeine alone, before or after exercise, abolished the effect of PEH [86–89]. The ingestion of two and three doses of coffee completely blunts the PEH, while one dose results in partial elimination of the PEH [89]. The magnitude of the BP reduction after exercise sessions is directly related to the pre-intervention BP of participants. Future studies on this issue are warranted.

Summary

In accordance with the hypertension evidence syntheses, only aerobic exercise session performed alone demonstrates sustained reductions (12 hours) in diastolic blood pressure. The studies assessing resistance training programs are needed, since reductions in diastolic BP were found with a greater number of resistance exercises, although these exercises also led to a minor decrease in systolic BP. It is possible that the residual fatigue resulting from high-intensity resistance exercise elevates the cardiovascular stress during daily activities of the participants, impairing the potential PEH of continuous aerobic exercise when performed simultaneously with resistance exercise. Since the combination of resistance and aerobic exercises is the most effective strategy to improve functional independence in the elderly population, future studies investigating additional concurrent training strategies are encouraged in order to increase the observed effects and possibly reveal underlying PEH mechanisms of this intervention in hypertensives. The food and selected substances may collaborate with physical exercise to increase the hypotensive response; that is, the synergy of these two interventions may improve the hypotensive results. Different food should be investigated regarding the power of association with exercise programs or sessions to reduce BP.

References

1. World Health Organization 2013. http://www.who.int/gho/ncd/risk_factors/blood_pressure_prevalence/en/.
2. Benjamin EJ, Blaha MJ, Chiuve SE, Cushman M, Das RS, Deo R, de Ferranti SD, Floyd J, Fornage M, Gillespie C, sasi CR, Jiménez MC, Jordan JC, Judd SE, Lackland D, Lichtman JH, Lisabeth L, Liu S, Longenecker CT, Mackey RH, Matsushita K, Mozaffarian D, Mussolino ME, Nasir K, Neumar RW, Palaniappan L, Pandey DK, Thiagarajan RR, Reeves MJ, Ritchey M, Rodriguez CJ, Roth GA, Rosamond WD, Sasson C, Towfighi A, Tsao CW, Turner MB, Virani SS, Voeks JH, Willey JZ, Wilkins JT, Wu JHY, Alger HM, Wong SS, Muntner P, On behalf of the American Heart Association Statistics Committee and Stroke Statistics Subcommittee. Heart disease and stroke statistics- 2017 update: a report from the American Heart Association. Circulation. 2017;135:e146–603.
3. Egan BM, Li J, Hutchison FN, Ferdinand KC. Hypertension in the United States, 1999 to 2012: progress toward healthy people 2020 goals. Circulation. 2014;130:1692–9.
4. Yeung PK, Kolathuru SS, Mohammadizadeh S, Akhoundi F, Linderfield B. Adenosine 50-triphosphate metabolism in red blood cells as a potential biomarker for post-exercise hypotension and a drug target for cardiovascular protection. Metabolites. 2018;8:30.
5. Fitzgerald W. Labile hypertension and jogging: new diagnostic tool or spurious discovery? BMJ (Clin Res Ed). 1981;282:542–4.
6. Kenney MJ, Seals DR. Postexercise hypotension. Key features, mechanisms, and clinical significance. Hypertension. 1993;22:653–64.
7. Pescatello LS, MacDonald HV, Ash GI, Lamberti LM, Farquhar WB, Arena R, Johnson BT. Assessing the existing professional exercise recommendations for hypertension: a review and recommendations for future research priorities. Mayo Clin Proc. 2015;90:801–12.
8. Pescatello LS, MacDonald HV, Lamberti L, Johnson BT. Exercise for hypertension: a prescription update integrating existing recommendations with emerging research. Curr Hypertens Rep. 2015;17:87.
9. Pescatello LS, Kulikowich JM. The aftereffects of dynamic exercise on ambulatory blood pressure. Med Sci Sports Exerc. 2001;33:1855–61.
10. Thompson PD, Crouse SF, Goodpaster B, Kelley D, Moyna N, Pescatello L. The acute versus the chronic response to exercise. Med Sci Sports Exerc. 2001;33 Suppl 6:S438–45; discussion S452–3.
11. Collier SR, Kanaley JA, Carhart R Jr, Frechette V, Tobin MM, Hall AK, Luckenbaugh AN, Fernhall B. Effect of 4 weeks of aerobic or resistance exercise training on arterial stiffness, blood flow and blood pressure in pre- and stage-1 hypertensives. J Hum Hypertens. 2008;22:678–86.
12. Pescatello LS, Franklin BA, Fagard R, Farquhar WB, Kelley GA, Ray CA, American College of Sports Medicine. American College of Sports Medicine position stand. Exercise and hypertension. Med Sci Sports Exerc. 2004;36:533–53.

13. Green DJ, Dawson EA, Groenewoud HM, Jones HJ, Thijssen DH. Is flow-mediated dilation nitric oxide mediated?: a meta-analysis. Hypertension. 2014;63:376–82.
14. Bruneau ML Jr, Johnson BT, Huedo-Medina TB, Larson KA, Ash GI, Pescatello LS. The blood pressure response to acute and chronic aerobic exercise: a meta-analysis of candidate gene association studies. J Sci Med Sport. 2016;19:424–31.
15. Stamler R. Implications of the INTERSALT study. Hypertension. 1991;17:I16–20.
16. Moraes MR, Bacurau RF, Simoes HG, Campbell CS, Pudo MA, Wasinski F, Pesquero JB, Wurtele M, Araujo RC. Effect of 12 weeks of resistance exercise on post-exercise hypotension in stage 1 hypertensive individuals. J Hum Hypertens. 2012;26:533–9.
17. Carpio-Rivera E, Moncada-Jiménez J, Salazar-Rojas W, Solera-Herrera A. Acute effects of exercise on blood pressure: a meta-analytic investigation. Arq Bras Cardiol. 2016;106:422–33.
18. Hagberg JM, Ferrell RE, Dengel DR, Wilund KR. Exercise training-induced blood pressure and plasma lipid improvements in hypertensives may be genotype dependent. Hypertension. 1999;34:18–23.
19. Hagberg JM, Park JJ, Brown MD. The role of exercise training in the treatment of hypertension: an update. Sports Med. 2000;30:193–206.
20. Rankinen T, Gagnon J, Perusse L, Chagnon YC, Rice T, Leon AS, Skinner JS, Wilmore JH, Rao DC, Bouchard C. AGT M235T and ACE ID polymorphisms and exercise blood pressure in the HERITAGE Family Study. Am J Physiol Heart Circ Physiol. 2000;279:H368–74.
21. Rankinen T, Rice T, Perusse L, Chagnon YC, Gagnon J, Leon AS, Skinner JS, Wilmore JH, Rao DC, Bouchard C. NOS3 Glu298Asp genotype and blood pressure response to endurance training: the HERITAGE family study. Hypertension. 2000;36:885–9.
22. Rankinen T, Rice T, Leon AS, Skinner JS, Wilmore JH, Rao DC, Bouchard C. G protein beta 3 polymorphism and hemodynamic and body composition phenotypes in the HERITAGE Family Study. Physiol Genomics. 2002;8:151–7.
23. Rankinen T, Church T, Rice T, Markward N, Leon AS, Rao DC, Skinner JS, Blair SN, Bouchard C. Effect of endothelin 1 genotype on blood pressure is dependent on physical activity or fitness levels. Hypertension. 2007;50:1120–5.
24. Rice T, An P, Gagnon J, Leon AS, Skinner JS, Wilmore JH, Bouchard C, Rao DC. Heritability of HR and BP response to exercise training in the HERITAGE Family Study. Med Sci Sports Exerc. 2002;34:972–9.
25. Bouchard C, Rankinen T. Individual differences in response to regular physical activity. Med Sci Sports Exerc. 2001;33 Suppl 6:S446–51; discussion S452–3.
26. Anunciação PG. Polito MD. A review on post-exercise hypotension in hypertensive individuals. Arq Bras Cardiol. 2011;96:e100–9.
27. Halliwill JR. Mechanisms and clinical implications of post-exercise hypotension in humans. Exerc Sport Sci Rev. 2001;29:65–70.
28. Rao SP, Collins HL, Dicarlo SE. Postexercise alpha-adrenergic receptor hyporesponsiveness in hypertensive rats is due to nitric oxide. Am J Physiol Regul Integr Comp Physiol. 2002;282:R960–8.
29. Boushel R, Langberg H, Gemmer C, Olesen J, Crameri R, Scheede C, Sander M, Kjaer M. Combined inhibition of nitric oxide and prostaglandins reduces human skeletal muscle blood flow during exercise. J Physiol. 2002;543(Pt 2):691–8.
30. Mortensen SP, Nyberg M, Thaning P, Saltin B, Hellsten Y. Adenosine contributes to blood flow regulation in the exercising human leg by increasing prostaglandin and nitric oxide formation. Hypertension. 2009;53:993–9.
31. Zafeiridis A. Mechanisms and exercise characteristics influencing postexercise hypotension. Br J Med Med Res. 2014;4:5699–714.
32. Chen C-Y, Bonham AC. Postexercise hypotension: central mechanisms. Exerc Sport Sci Rev. 2010;38:122–7.
33. Powers SK, Ji LL, Leeuwenburgh C. Exercise training–induced alterations in skeletal muscle antioxidant capacity: a brief review. Med Sci Sports Exerc. 1999;31:987–97.

34. Dudzinska W, Lubkowska A, Dolegowska B, Safranow K, Jakubowska K. Adenine, guanine and pyridine nucleotides in blood during physical exercise and restitution in healthy subjects. Eur J Appl Physiol. 2010;110:1155–62.
35. Halliwill JR, Buck TM, Lacewell AN, Romero SA. Postexercise hypotension and sustained postexercise vasodilatation: what happens after we exercise? Exp Physiol. 2013;98:7–18.
36. Ray CA, Carrasco DI. Isometric handgrip training reduces arterial pressure at rest without changes in sympathetic nerve activity. Am J Physiol Heart Circ Physiol. 2000;279:H245–9.
37. Clifford PS, Hellsten Y. Vasodilatory mechanisms in contracting skeletal muscle. J Appl Physiol. 1985;97:393–403.
38. Melo CM, AlencarFilho AC, Tinucci T, Mion D Jr, Forjaz CL. Postexercise hypotension induced by low-intensity resistance exercise in hypertensive women receiving captopril. Blood Press Monit. 2006;11:183–9.
39. Fisher MM. The effect of resistance exercise on recovery blood pressure in normotensive and borderline hypertensive women. J Strength Cond Res. 2001;15:210–6.
40. Hardy DO, Tucker LA. The effects of a single bout of strength training on ambulatory blood pressure levels in 24 mildly hypertensive men. Am J Health Promot. 1998;13:69–72.
41. Moraes MR, Bacurau RF, Ramalho JD, Reis FC, Casarini DE, Chagas JR, et al. Increase in kinins on post-exercise hypotension in normotensive and hypertensive volunteers. Biol Chem. 2007;388:533–40.
42. Mediano MFFP, Paravidino V, Simão R, Pontes FL, Polito MD. Subacute behavior of the blood pressure after power training in controlled hypertensive individuals. Rev Bras Med Esporte. 2005;11:337–40.
43. BrandaoRondon MU, Alves MJ, Braga AM, et al. Postexercise blood pressure reduction in elderly hypertensive patients. J Am Coll Cardiol. 2002;39:676–82.
44. Taylor-Tolbert NS, Dengel DR, Brown MD, et al. Ambulatory blood pressure after acute exercise in older men with essential hypertension. Am J Hypertens. 2000;13:44–51.
45. Brito Ade F, de Oliveira CV, Brasileiro-Santos Mdo S, Santos Ada C. Resistance exercise with different volumes: blood pressure response and forearm blood flow in the hypertensive elderly. Clin Interv Aging. 2014;9:2151–8.
46. Keese F, Farinatti P, Pescatello L, Monteiro W. A comparison of the immediate effects of resistance, aerobic, and concurrent exercise on postexercise hypotension. J Strength Cond Res. 2011;25:1429–36.
47. Ruiz RJ, Simao R, Saccomani MG, Casonatto J, Alexander JL, Rhea M, Polito MD. Isolated and combined effects of aerobic and strength exercise on post-exercise blood pressure and cardiac vagal reactivation in normotensive men. J Strength Cond Res. 2011;25:640–5.
48. Teixeira L, Ritti-Dias RM, Tinucci T, Mion Junior D, Forjaz CL. Post-concurrent exercise hemodynamics and cardiac autonomic modulation. Eur J Appl Physiol. 2011;111:2069–78.
49. Brito Ade F, de Oliveira CV, Santos MDS, Santos Ada C. High-intensity exercise promotes postexercise hypotension greater than moderate intensity in elderly hypertensive individuals. Clin Physiol Funct Imag. 2014;34:126–32.
50. de FreitasBrito A, Brasileiro-Santos MDS, Coutinho de Oliveira CV, Sarmento da Nóbrega TK, Lúcia de MoraesForjaz C, da Cruz Santos A. High-intensity resistance exercise promotes postexercise hypotension greater than moderate intensity and affects cardiac autonomic responses in women who are hypertensive. J Strength Cond Res. 2015;29:3486–93.
51. de Freitas Brito A, Brasileiro-Santos MDS, de Coutinho, Oliveira CV, de Cruz Santos A. Postexercise hypotension is volume-dependent in hypertensives: autonomic and forearm blood responses. J Strength Cond Res. 2018; https://doi.org/10.1519/JSC.0000000000001735.
52. Joubert DP, Granados JZ, Oliver JM, Noack BL, Grandjean PW, Woodman CR, Riechman SE, Crouse SF. An acute bout of aquatic treadmill exercise induces greater improvements in endothelial function and post-exercise hypotension than land treadmill exercise: a crossover study. Am J Phys Med Rehabil. 2018; https://doi.org/10.1097/PHM.0000000000000923.
53. Chen YM. Perceived barriers to physical activity among older adults residing in long-term care institutions. J Clin Nurs. 2010;19:432–9.

54. Millar PJ, McGowan CL, Cornelissen VA, Araujo CG, Swaine IL. Evidence for the role of isometric exercise training in reducing blood pressure: potential mechanisms and future directions. Sports Med. 2014;44:345–56.
55. Badrov MB, Horton S, Millar PJ, McGowan CL. Cardiovascular stress reactivity tasks successfully predict the hypotensive response of isometric handgrip training in hypertensives. Psychophysiology. 2013;50:407–14.
56. Carlson DJ, Dieberg G, Hess NC, Millar PJ, Smart NA. Isometric exercise training for blood pressure management: a systematic review and meta-analysis. Mayo Clin Proc. 2014;89:327–34.
57. McGowan CL, Visocchi A, Faulkner M, Verduyn R, Rakobowchuk M, Levy AS, McCartney N, MacDonald MJ. Isometric handgrip training improves local flow-mediated dilation in medicated hypertensives. Eur J Appl Physiol. 2007;99:227–34.
58. Taylor AC, McCartney N, Kamath MV, Wiley RL. Isometric training lowers resting blood pressure and modulates autonomic control. Med Sci Sports Ecerc. 2003;35:251–6.
59. Souza LR, Vicente JB, Melo GR, Moraes VC, Olher RR, Sousa IC, Peruchi LH, Neves RV, Rosa TS, Ferreira AP, Moraes MR. Acute hypotension after moderate-intensity handgrip exercise in hypertensive elderly people. J Strength Cond Res. 2018; https://doi.org/10.1519/JSC.0000000000002460.
60. Olher RRV, Bocalini DS, Bacurau RF, Rodriguez D, Figueira A Jr, Pontes FL Jr, Navarro F, Simões HG, Araujo RC, Moraes MR. Isometric handgrip does not elicit cardiovascular overload or post-exercise hypotension in hypertensive older women. Clin Interv Aging. 2013;8:649–55.
61. Cadore EL, Pinto RS, Bottaro M, Izquierdo M. Strength and endurance training prescription in healthy and frail elderly. Aging Dis. 2014;5:183–95.
62. Ferrari R, Umpierre D, Vogel G, Vieira PJC, Santos LP, de Mello RB, Tanaka H, Fuchs SC. Effects of concurrent and aerobic exercises on postexercise hypotension in elderly hypertensive men. Exp Gerontol. 2017;98:1–7.
63. Jones H, George K, Edwards B, Atkinson G. Is the magnitude of acute post-exercise hypotension mediated by exercise intensity or total work done? Eur J Appl Physiol. 2007;102:33–40.
64. Hamer M. The anti-hypertensive effects of exercise: integrating acute and chronic mechanisms. Sports Med. 2006;36:109–16.
65. Thijssen DH, Dawson EA, van den Munckhof IC, Birk GK, Timothy Cable N, Green DJ. Local and systemic effects of leg cycling training on arterial wall thickness in healthy humans. Atherosclerosis. 2013;229:282–6.
66. Miyai N, Shiozaki M, Yabu M, Utsumi M, Morioka I, Miyashita K, et al. Increased mean arterial pressure response to dynamic exercise in normotensive subjects with multiple metabolic risk factors. Hypertens Res. 2013;36:534–9.
67. Rahmouni K, Correia ML, Haynes WG, Mark AL. Obesity-associated hypertension: new insights into mechanisms. Hypertension. 2005;45:9–14.
68. Schoenenberger AW, Schoenenberger-Berzins R, Suter PM, Erne P. Effects of weight on blood pressure at rest and during exercise. Hypertens Res. 2013;36:1045–50.
69. Canuto PM, Nogueira ID, Cunha ES, Ferreira GM, Pinto KM, Costa FA, Nogueira PA. Influence of resistance training performed at different intensities and same work volume over BP of elderly hypertensive female patients. Rev Bras Med Esporte. 2011;17:246–9.
70. Brito AF, Oliveira CVC, Toscano LT, Silva AS. Supplements and foods with potential reduction of blood pressure in prehypertensive and hypertensive subjects: a systematic review. ISRN Hypertension. 2013;2013:1–15.
71. Leibowitz A, Faltin Z, Perl A, Eshdat Y, Hagay Y, Peleg E, Grossman E. Red grape berry–cultured cells reduce blood pressure in rats with metabolic-like syndrome. Eur J Nutr. 2014;53:973–80.
72. Patki G, Allam FH, Atrooz F, Dao AT, Solanki N, Chugh G, Asghar M, Jafri F, Bohat R, Alkadhi KA, Salim S. Grape powder intake prevents ovariectomy-induced anxiety-like behavior, memory impairment and high blood pressure in female Wistar rats. PLoS One. 2013;8:e74522.

73. Park YK, Kim JS, Kang MH. Concord grape juice supplementation reduces blood pressure in Korean hypertensive men: double-blind, placebo controlled intervention trial. Biofactors. 2004;22:145–7.
74. Park YK, Lee SH, Park E, Kim JS, Kang MH. Changes in antioxidant status, blood pressure, and lymphocyte DNA damage from grape juice supplementation. Ann N Y Acad Sci. 2009;1171:385–90.
75. Belcaro G, Ledda A, Hu S, Cesarone MR, Feragalli B, Dugall M. Grape seed procyanidins in pre- and mild hypertension: a registry study. Evid Based Complement Alternat Med. 2013;2013:1–15.
76. Dohadwala MM, Vita JA. Grapes and cardiovascular disease. J Nutr. 2009;139:1788S–93S.
77. Noguer MA, Cerezo AB, Navarro ED, Garcia-Parrilla MC. Intake of alcohol-free red wine modulates antioxidant enzyme activities in a human intervention study. Pharmacol Res. 2012;65:609–14.
78. Neto MM, da Silva TF, de Lima FF, Siqueira TMQ, Toscano LT, de Moura SKMSF, Silva AS. Whole red grape juice reduces blood pressure at rest and increases post-exercise hypotension. J Am Coll Nutr. 2017;36:533–40.
79. Guidry MA, Blanchard BE, Thompson PD, Maresh CM, Seip RL, Taylor AL, Pescatello LS. The influence of short and long duration on the blood pressure response to an acute bout of dynamic exercise. Am Heart J. 2006;151:1322.e5–12.
80. Monteiro MF, SobralFilho DC. Physical exercise and blood pressure control. Rev Bras Med Esporte. 2004;10:513–6.
81. Casonatto J, Polito MD. Post-exercise hypotension: a systematic review. Rev Bras Med Esporte. 2009;15:151–7.
82. Marques-Silvestre ACOM, Santos MSB, Oliveira AS, Silva FTM, Santos AC. Magnitude of hypotension after acute aerobic exercise: a systematic review of randomized trials. Motricidade. 2014;10:99–111.
83. Pardono E, Almeida MB, Bastos AA, Simões HG. Post-exercise hypotension: possible relationship with ethnic and genetic factors. Rev Bras Cineantropom Desempenho Hum. 2012;14:353–61.
84. Junior JFCR, Silva AS, Cardoso GA, Silvino VO, Martins MCC, Santos MAP. Androgenic-anabolic steroids inhibited post-exercise hypotension: a case control study. Braz J Phys Ther. 2018;22:77–81.
85. O'Keefe JH, Bhatti SK, Patil HR, DiNicolantonio JJ, Lucan SC, Lavie CJ. Effects of habitual coffee consumption on cardiometabolic disease, cardiovascular health, and all-cause mortality. J Am Coll Cardiol. 2013;62:1043–51.
86. Notarius CF, Morris BL, Floras JS. Caffeine attenuates early post-exercise hypotension in middle-aged subjects. Am J Hypertens. 2006;19:184–8.
87. Cazé RF, Franco GAM, Porpino SKP, Souza AA, Padilhas OP, Silva AS. Caffeine influence on blood pressure response to aerobic exercise in hypertensive subjects. Rev Bras Med Esporte. 2010;16:324–8.
88. Nóbrega TKS, Moura Junior JS, Alves NFB, Santos AC, Silva AS. A ingestão de café abole a hipotensão induzida porexercício aeróbio: um estudopiloto. Revista da EducaçâoFísica/UEM. Maringá. 2011;22:601–12.
89. Souza AA, Silva RS, Silva TF, Tavares RL, Silva AS. Influence of different doses of coffee on post-exercise blood pressure response. Am J Cardiovasc Dis. 2016;6:146–52.

Nocturnal Hypotension

6

Kannayiram Alagiakrishnan

Introduction

Blood pressure (BP) normally decreases during the night. It is usually lower during sleep at nighttime by 10–20%. Based on the day night blood pressure ratio from 24-hour ambulatory blood pressure recordings, normal BP dip or otherwise defined as dipper is the ratio ≤0.9 and >0.8, whereas extreme dippers or nocturnal hypotension on the night-day blood pressure is the ratio ≤0.8. It has been 30 years since the dipping phenomenon was first coined by O'Brien and colleagues [1]. In healthy individuals, nighttime BP decreases by 10–20% and increases promptly on waking. However, certain abnormal diurnal variation patterns have been described in which the nocturnal fall of BP may be more than 20% called extreme dippers or nocturnal hypotension.

Nocturnal Hypotension and Cardiac Morbidities

Coronary Artery Disease (CAD)

Extreme dippers due to pharmacological reduction were associated with increase in the number and duration of cardiac ischemic episodes in hypertensive subjects [2]. In hypertensive subjects with no history of coronary artery disease, extreme dipper subjects had greater arterial stiffness than in dippers, which caused impaired coronary artery microcirculation and increased risk of myocardial ischemia [3]. However Verdecchia et al. in their longitudinal study over 8 years period did not find a statistically significant difference in cardiovascular risk between extreme dippers and dippers after correcting for co-variates in the study. Also, a greater morning BP surge,

K. Alagiakrishnan (✉)
Division of Geriatric Medicine, University of Alberta, Edmonton, AB, Canada

© Springer Nature Switzerland AG 2020
K. Alagiakrishnan, M. Banach (eds.), *Hypotensive Syndromes in Geriatric Patients*, https://doi.org/10.1007/978-3-030-30332-7_6

either expressed as sleep-trough or preawakening surge, did not predict a greater cardiovascular risk in this study [4].

Left Ventricular Hypertrophy (LVH)

In a cardiac MRI study Rodrigues et al. showed a larger nocturnal blood drop was associated with more LVH. Left ventricular mass was significantly higher for extreme dippers than dippers after correction for co-variates (100 ± 6 g/m^2 vs 79 ± 3 g/m^2, $P = 0.004$) [5].

Nocturnal Hypotension and Cerebrovascular Disease (CVD)

Kario et al. showed that excessive reductions in nighttime systolic BP values can contribute to silent cerebral infarction [6, 7]. Extreme nocturnal fall in BP can lead to more cerebral ischemia, resulting in Binswanger's lesions, cerebral lacunae, and periventricular hyperlucencies were seen on magnetic resonance imaging of the brain.

Nocturnal Hypotension and Eye Diseases

Glaucoma

Nocturnal hypotension is associated with visual loss from glaucoma, however, has yielded controversial results [8, 9]. However in a study with Normal Tension Glaucoma (NTG) patients who had ambulatory blood pressure monitoring for 48 hours and visual field testing at baseline, 6 and 12 months, nocturnal hypotension was a significant predictor of visual field loss progression ($P <0.02$) [10]. In the recent Maracaibo Aging Study, extreme dippers significantly increased the risk of glaucomatous optic neuropathy [11].

Optic Ischemic Neuropathy

In older subjects acute optic neuropathy due to ischemia is common and is due to vascular insufficiency of the optic nerve [12]. Role of nocturnal arterial hypotension in nonarteritic anterior ischemic optic neuropathy (NAION) has been discussed [13]. In 1994, Hayreh et al. in their study showed evidence, not only for NAION but also for NTG (normal tension glaucoma) and POAG (primary open angle glaucoma). Significant association between progressive visual field deterioration and nocturnal hypotension was seen, particularly when patients took antihypertensive medications in the evening or at bedtime [14]. Nocturnal hypotension can also lead to anterior ischemic optic neuropathy (AION) and it can present as visual loss on awakening. Nocturnal hypotension can impair optic disc circulation. Systemic hypertension may have impaired autoregulation of optic disc circulation and nocturnal hypotension by pathophysiological basis or by aggressive nighttime antihypertensive therapy may lead to ischemic injuries [15].

Nocturnal Hypotension and Blood Pressure Dysregulation (Postural Hypertension and Early Morning Surge)

In persons prone to extreme dipping, the decline in nocturnal BP is typically >20% for both Systolic blood pressure (SBP) and Diastolic blood pressure (DBP). Extreme dipping has been associated with postural hypertension and increased risk of silent cerebrovascular disease [16, 17]. In subjects who are having lower nocturnal blood pressure, the more pronounced is the morning surge in blood pressure [18].

Pathophysiology of Nocturnal Hypotension

Circadian rhythm of blood pressure is regulated by autonomic nervous system and genetic alternations may also play a role. Blood pressure changes happen with different sleep stages. During deep NREM sleep, sympathetic nervous system activity decreases than during wakefulness and increases in REM sleep. Blood pressure declines with NREM sleep and increases with REM sleep. With excessive nighttime BP drop (extreme dippers or nocturnal hypotension), there has been more pronounced morning surge with cerebral, coronary, and ophthalmic ischemic changes [19–21]. Cohen et al., in their meta-analysis study of 83,929 subjects, found a 40% increase of myocardial infarction in the morning hours when compared with the rest of the day [22]. Similarly Elliot et al. in their meta-analysis of 11,816 subjects found a 49% increase in the risk of stroke in the morning hours when compared with rest of the day [23]. Both these events could be due to early morning surge in BP. The increase in cardiovascular and cerebrovascular adverse events observed during the morning is associated with a pronounced rise in plasma catecholamine and cortisol levels. This increases the heart rate and blood pressure and enhances the myocardial oxygen demand and causes also a hypercoagulable state. This can also increase vascular tone and increase in blood viscosity and platelet aggregability, which can lead to ischemic events [24].

Measurement of Nocturnal Hypotension

Nocturnal hypotension can be measured by 24-hour ambulatory BP measurement (24-hour ABPM) [25]. ABPM is a form of automatic monitoring of blood pressure whereby measurements are serially taken over 24-hour period. ABPM was first developed in 1962 and subsequently modified by Skolow et al. in 1966 [26]. During the past five decades, there was development with new ABPM devices and is now widely used for routine clinical purposes. Evidence is accumulating that ABP measurements provide a better prediction of clinical outcome as compared with conventional clinic BP measurements [27]. Office BP measurement is not an ideal method for representing 24-hour blood pressure with its diurnal and nocturnal blood pressure variability compared with ambulatory blood pressure monitoring [28, 29]. Using ABPM, morning, daytime, nighttime, and average 24-hour BP levels can be measured. 24-hour ABPM was a better indicator of end organ damage than office measurement. ABPM method is now considered a gold standard for nocturnal hypotension measurement. Also ambulatory 24-hour BP monitoring is safe, relatively inexpensive and easy to obtain [30]. Current ABPM devices are automated, small and convenient, and non-invasive and can evaluate the BP over 24-hour period including during sleep and normal activities (Table 6.1).

Management of Nocturnal Hypotension

Some studies had shown that medication management of hypertension with certain antihypertensive medication can influence the circadian diurnal rhythm. In an Italian study, a short-acting angiotensin-converting enzyme inhibitor quinapril was administered after a placebo period either at 8 am or 10 pm in a cross-over fashion. With 10 pm dosing, drop in blood pressure is more (10–15% additional drop) between 2 am and 6 am with an increased surge in BP between 6 and 8 am which might put the patients at risk for ischemic events [31].

Smoothness index is a measure that assesses the degree of 24-hour BP reduction in clinical trials of antihypertensive medication efficacy, which has been correlated with hypertension-associated target organ damage. Certain antihypertensive agents like telmisartan and amlodipine have been shown to provide a smooth 24-hour BP control, including the early morning period [32, 33]. Controlled-onset extended-release (COER) verapamil, taken in the evening, due to its water-soluble delay coating has its antihypertensive effect 4–5 hours after ingestion, avoiding the nighttime trough in BP, and releases the medication in the early morning hours to help with the surge in BP [34]. This effect was studied in 29 healthy men after 5 days of oral

Table 6.1 Nighttime and early morning BP measurements calculations

1. Nighttime BP dipping parameters [39]
(a) Nighttime BP dipping (%) was calculated as (1 − SBP/average daytime SBP) × 100.
Subgroup classification based on nighttime dipping was defined as
Extreme dipper: >20%.
Dipper: ≤20%, >10%.
Non-dipper: ≤10%, >0%.
Riser: ≤0%.
(b) Night/day BP ratios
0.8 indicated an extreme dipper.
>0.8 to 0.9 indicated a dipper.
>0.9 to 1.0 indicated a non-dipper.
>1.0 indicated a reverse dipper.
2. Morning BP surge (MBPS) parameters [6, 40].
Prewakening MBPS: mean morning SBP for 2 hours after awakening-preawake SBP (2-hour average before awakening).
Sleep-trough MBPS: The difference between the mean systolic BP (SBP) over 2 hours following the awakening and the average of three BP values centered on the lowest nocturnal BP.

COER verapamil dosing at 10 pm. Plasma levels of the medication were found to be low during sleep and peaked during the early morning hours. This could avoid the exacerbation of the nocturnal blood pressure drop with untoward ischemic changes as well as the early morning surge with untoward catastrophic cardiovascular events [35]. But CONVINCE trial, showed the effectiveness of calcium channel blocker in reducing cardiovascular events was similar to diuretic or beta blocker treatment [36]. However a study by Kwon et al. showed amlodipine has better diurnal variation in blood pressure with better control on morning surge [37]. The effects of long-acting dihydropyridine calcium channel blockers have been shown to reduce not only daytime, but also nighttime and morning BP. This also helps to restore abnormal nocturnal dipping status toward a normal dipping pattern in hypertensive patients [38].

References

1. O'Brien E, Sheridan J, O'Malley K. Dippers and non-dippers. Lancet. 1988;2:397.
2. Pierdomenico SD, Bucci A, Costantini F, et al. Circadian blood pressure changes and myocardial ischemia in hypertensive patients with coronary artery disease. J Am Coll Cardiol. 1998;31:1627–34.
3. Amah G, Quardani R, Pasteur-Rousseau A, et al. Extreme-dipper profile, increased aortic stiffness, and impaired subendocardial viability in hypertension. Am J Hypertens. 2017;30(4):417–26.
4. Verdecchia P, Angeli F, Mazzotta G, et al. Day-night dip and early-morning surge in blood pressure in hypertension: prognostic implications. Hypertension. 2012;60:34–42.
5. Rodrigues JCL, Amadu AM, Dastidar GA, et al. Noctural dipping status and left ventricular hypertrophy: a cardiac magnetic resonance imaging study. J Clin Hypertens. 2018;20(4):784–93.
6. Kario K, Pickering TG, Umeda Y, et al. Morning surge in blood pressure as a predictor of silent and clinical cerebrovascular disease in elderly hypertensives: a prospective study. Circulation. 2003;107:1401–6.
7. Kario K, Matsuo T, Kobayashi H, et al. Nocturnal fall of blood pressure and silent cerebrovascular damage in elderly hypertensive patients. Advanced silent cerebrovascular damage in extreme dippers. Hypertension. 1996;27:130–5.
8. Graham L, Drance M, Wijsman K, et al. Ambulatory blood pressure monitoring in glaucoma. The nocturnal dip. Ophthalmology. 1995;102:61–9.
9. Collignon N, Dewe W, Guillaume S, et al. Ambulatory blood pressure monitoring in glaucoma patients, the nocturnal systolic dip and its relationship with disease progression. Int Ophthalmol. 1998;22:19–25.
10. Charlson ME, deMoraes CG, Link A, et al. Nocturnal systemic hypotension increases the risk of glaucoma progression. Ophthalmology. 2014;121:204–12.
11. Melgarejo JD, Lee JH, Petitto M. Glaucomatous optic neuropathy associated with nocturnal dip in blood pressure. Findings from the Maracaibo Aging Study. Ophthalmology. 2018;125:807–14.
12. Biousse V, Newman NJ. Ischemic optic neuropathies. N Engl J Med. 2015;372:2428–36.
13. Cestari DM, Arnold A. Does nocturnal hypotension play a causal role in nonarteritic anterior ischemic optic neuropathy? J Neuroophthalmol. 2016;36:329–33.
14. Hayreh SS, Zimmerman MB, Podhajsky P, et al. Nocturnal arterial hypotension and its role in optic nerve head and ocular ischemic disorders. Am J Ophthalmol. 1994;117:603–24.

15. Hayreh SS, Podhajsky PA, Zimmerman B. Role of nocturnal arterial hypotension in optic nerve head ischemic disorders. Ophthalmologica. 1999;213:76–96.
16. Xu T, Zhang YQ, Tan XR. The dilemma of nocturnal blood pressure. J Clin Hypertens. 2012;14:787–91.
17. Kario K, Eguchi K, Nakagawa Y, et al. Relationship between extreme dippers and orthostatic hypertension in elderly hypertensive patients. Hypertension. 1998;31:77–82.
18. Kario K, Mitsuhashi T, Shimada K. Neurohumoral characteristics of older hypertensive patients with abnormal nocturnal blood pressure dipping. Am J Hypertens. 2002;15:531–7.
19. Hermida RC, Ayala DE, Portaluppi F. Circadian variation of blood pressure: the basis for the chronotherapy of hypertension. Adv Drug Deliv Rev. 2007;59:904–22.
20. Douna LG, GumZ ML. Circadian clock- mediated regulation of blood pressure. Free Radic Biol Med. 2018;119:108–14.
21. Alagiakrishnan K, Masaki K, Schatz I, et al. Blood pressure dysregulation syndrome: the case for control throughout the circadian cycle. Geriatrics. 2001;56(3):50–6.
22. Cohen MC, Ruhtla KM, Lavery CE, et al. Meta-analysis of the morning excess of acute myocardial infarction and sudden cardiac death. Am J Cardiol. 1997;79:1512–6.
23. Elliott WJ. Circadian variation in the timing of stroke onset: a meta-analysis. Stroke. 1998;29:992–6.
24. Elliot WJ. Circadian variation in blood pressure. Implications for the elderly patient. AJH. 1999;12:43S–9S.
25. O'Brien E. Ambulatory blood pressure measurement-the case for implementation in primary care. Hypertension. 2008;51:1435–41.
26. Sokolow M, Werdegar D, Kain H, et al. Relationship between level of blood pressure measured casually and by portable recorders and severity of complications in essential hypertension. Circulation. 1966;34:279–98.
27. Verdecchia P, Schillaci G, Borgioni C, et al. Ambulatory pulse pressure. A potent predictor of total cardiovascular risk in hypertension. Hypertension. 1998;32:983–8.
28. Parati G. Blood pressure variability: its measurement and significance in hypertension. J Hypertens Suppl. 2005;23:S19–25.
29. Hodgkinson J, Mant J, Martin U, et al. Relative effectiveness of clinic and home blood pressure monitoring compared with ambulatory blood pressure monitoring in diagnosis of hypertension: systematic review. BMJ. 2011;342:d3621.
30. Thomas GP, Daichi S, Haas D. Ambulatory blood-pressure monitoring. N Engl J Med. 2006;354:2368–74.
31. Palatini P. Can an angiotensin-converting enzyme inhibitor with a short half-life effectively lower blood pressure for 24 hours? Am Heart J. 1992;123:1421–5.
32. Redon J. The importance of 24-hour ambulatory blood pressure monitoring in patients at risk of cardiovascular events. High Blood Press Cardiovasc Prev. 2013;20(1):13–8.
33. Dahlof B, Sever PS, Poulter NR, et al. Prevention of cardiovascular events with an antihypertensive regimen of amlodipine adding perindopril as required versus atenolol adding bendroflumethiazide as required, in the Anglo-Scandinavian Cardiac Outcomes Trial-Blood Pressure Lowering Arm (ASCOT-BPLA): a multicentre randomised controlled trial. Lancet. 2005;366:895–906.
34. Gupta SK, Yih BM, Atkinson L, et al. The effect of food, time of dosing, and body position on the pharmacokinetics and pharmacodynamic of verapamil and norverapamil. J Clin Pharmacol. 1995;35:1083–93.
35. White WB, Black HR, Weber MA, et al. Comparison of effects of controlled onset extended release verapamil at bedtime and nifedipine gastrointestinal therapeutic system on arising on early morning blood pressure, heart rate, and the heart rate-blood pressure product. Am J Cardiol. 1998;81:424–31.
36. Black RH, Elliot WJ, Grandits G, et al. Principal results of the controlled onset Verapamil Investigation of Cardiovascualr End Points (CONVINCE) trial. JAMA. 2003;289(16):2073–89.

37. Kwon HM, Shin JW, Lim JS, et al. Comparison of the effects of amlodipine and losartan on blood pressure and diurnal variation in hypertensive stroke patients: a prospective, randomized, double-blind, comparative parallel study. Clin Ther. 2013;35(12):1975–82.
38. Eguchi K. 24 hour perfect BP-lowering therapy using long-acting dihydropyridine calcium channel blockers. Nihon Rinsho. 2014;72(8):1461–5.
39. Fagard R, Thijs L, Staessen JA, et al. Night and day blood pressure ratio and dipping pattern as predictors of death and cardiovascular events in hypertension. J Hum Hypertens. 2009;23:645–53.
40. Shimada K, Kario K, Umeda Y, et al. Early morning surge in blood pressure. Blood Press Monit. 2001;6:349–53.

Non-pharmacological Management of Hypotensive Syndromes

7

Kannayiram Alagiakrishnan

Introduction

Non-pharmacological measures are the first line of management for different hypotensive syndromes, and if necessary, one should add pharmacological management. There are many non-pharmacological therapies, and education of these approaches by healthcare professionals to patients is important. Non-pharmacological approaches should be considered in all patients with asymptomatic or symptomatic hypotensive syndromes (Table 7.1).

Orthostatic Hypotension

Educating the Patient

In orthostatic hypotension (OH), discussing how to avoid precipitating factors like prolonged bed rest is important. Factors that may precipitate or worsen OH like hot baths or showers, sudden move from the lying to standing position, alcohol intake, straining especially with breath holding (Valsalva maneuver), and precautions to prevent it should be discussed in detail. Teaching in detail about these triggering situations is very important [1].

Lifestyle Modifications

Patient should understand that OH tends to be worst in the morning. They should avoid quick postural changes from lying or sitting position to standing position. Hot

K. Alagiakrishnan (✉)
Division of Geriatric Medicine, University of Alberta, Edmonton, AB, Canada

© Springer Nature Switzerland AG 2020
K. Alagiakrishnan, M. Banach (eds.), *Hypotensive Syndromes in Geriatric Patients*, https://doi.org/10.1007/978-3-030-30332-7_7

Table 7.1 Non-pharmacological measures in different hypotensive syndromes

Orthostatic Hypotension
Patient education
Avoiding warm environment
Avoiding excessive alcohol use
Drinking fluids up to 1.5–2 l
Avoiding straining activity
Standing-up slowly from lying position
Squatting, leg crossing
Increasing salt intake
Waist-high compression stockings
Sleeping in the head-up position
Postprandial Hypotension
Multiple small meals of protein and fat
Avoiding alcohol with meals
Walking exercise after meals
Cold rather than warm meals
Vasovagal Syncope
Patient education
Avoiding triggers
Increasing salt and water intake
Physical countermeasures
Carotid Sinus Hypersensitivity
Avoiding vigorous head turning
Avoiding tight shirt collars
Increasing salt and water intake
Exercise-Induced Hypotension
Performing exercise in sitting or supine positions, as exercising in the upright position worsens hypotension
Avoiding food intake before exercise
Nocturnal Hypotension
Extreme-dipping status of nocturnal BP is closely associated with excessive morning BP surge and orthostatic hypertension. So slow rise from lying position may be helpful.

temperature is known to provoke or worsen OH. Autonomic nervous system cardio-vascular adaptation plays a role in homeostatic control of body temperature [2]. Avoiding overheated rooms and hot baths or saunas is advisable.

Patients need to be more vigilant about hot environments during summer and should avoid hot baths and hot rooms. Pathak et al. in their study in 2004, during the heat wave in France, found heat-related morbidity was higher in elderly subjects with neurogenic OH [3]. In a small study, Petrofsy et al. found diabetic patients reported more drop in OH by using tilt table testing in a hot environment warm room (42 degrees Celsius) than at neutral temperature room (22 degrees Celsius) [4].

As physical deconditioning can cause or worsen OH, exercise should be encouraged. Physical maneuvers like leg crossing and tensing of the muscles of the legs and arms may raise blood pressure (BP). Even small increase in BP may prevent symptoms of presyncope and syncope [5]. A study showed crossing legs on standing increases venous return and peripheral resistance, thereby helping to reduce the orthostatic drop in BP [6].

In subjects with OH, alcohol should be avoided or used minimally as it can cause diuresis and volume loss by suppressing anti-diuretic hormone, as well as cause vasodilatation and worsen orthostatic drop in blood pressure [7]. Elevating the head of the bed by 30 degrees tilt during sleep can limit supine hypertension and reduce early morning postural hypotension. The possible mechanism that can happen is by stimulating the carotid and aortic baroreceptors as well as the renin angiotensin system.

Adequate Fluid Intake

Drinking additional water has an acute pressor effect in patient with OH. Rehydration, oropharyngeal activation, gastric dilatation, osmosensitivite mechanisms, all cause a rise in sympathetic activity which has been implicated in the pressor response with water drinking [8–10]. In a study by Jordan et al. in older subjects when they drank 480 ml of water, there was a pressor effect by 11 mm Hg, and in these subjects, there was an increase in plasma norepinephrine levels [11] (Table 7.2).

Volume expansion by increasing sodium intake and fluid ingestion up to 2–2.5 l has been suggested. Urinary sodium excretion >170 mEq/24 h and urinary volume > 1500 ml indicate adequate fluid and salt intake [12–14]. In a case series study by Deguchi et al., drinking 350 ml of tap water demonstrated excellent pressor effects, which alleviated intractable OH in the early morning inpatients with MSA and the pressor effects were seen for seven successive days. In addition, there was also improvement of orthostatic symptoms. This intervention was useful even with combined OH and postprandial hypotension (PPH), and it reduced the blood pressure drop [15].

Table 7.2 Mechanisms of these non-pharmacological strategies in hypotensive syndromes

Cold water intake via a gastropressor response increases the sympathetic activity.
Raise the head end of bed during sleep diminish renal filtration and reduce nocturnal polyuria, and it also increases angiotensin II production, thus reducing risk of volume depletion in the morning.
Stockings that compress both legs and abdomen reduce venous pooling in the splanchnic and peripheral venous circulations.
Avoiding heat, alcohol intake prevents peripheral vasodilatation and consumption of small meals, which can prevent splanchnic vasodilatation.
Contraction of a group of muscles, leg crossing, toe raising, and bending at the waist transiently increase venous return and peripheral vascular resistance.

Salt Intake

A dietary intake of at least 2–3 g (37–55.5 mmol) of sodium per day has been suggested. In some patients with severe disease, higher salt intake may be recommended but should be weighed against the risk of volume overload with different comorbid conditions [12]. Restoration of plasma volume with salt tablets and water had been shown in a study of subjects after bed rest resulted in a zero rate of orthostatic hypotension [16].

Sleeping in the Head-Up Position

Studies have showed the effectiveness of sleeping in the head-up position (SHU) in OH [17]. However, an open RCT by Fan et al. showed SHU had variable effectiveness in elderly subjects [18]. Nocturnal polyuria causing intravascular volume depletion had been shown in autonomic failure patients [19]. Since the legs are below the heart position, a decrease in renal arterial pressure leads to activation of renin angiotensin with increasing angiotensin II production. It can also reduce the risk of volume depletion in the morning by reducing nocturnal polyuria [20].

Waist-High Compression Stockings

Therapies that help to reduce pooling in the periphery and in the splanchnic circulation by using compression stockings and abdominal binders might be helpful in the management of OH. Peripheral vascular disease should be ruled out before applying these devices [21–23].

In a recent study, Newton JL et al. compared the efficacy of different non-pharmacological measures in 25 older people (age 60–92 years) to determine cardiovascular responses to bolus water drinking, compression stockings, abdominal compression, and physical counter maneuvers, by measuring proportion of participants whose systolic blood pressure drop improved by $\geq$10 mm Hg. Among the non-pharmacological measures, the response rate to bolus water drinking was 56% (95% confidence interval [CI] 36.7–74.2), with standing SBP increasing by 12 mm Hg (95% CI 4–20), but none of these non-pharmacological interventions improved symptoms during standing. All the interventions in this study did not show any adverse events. This study showed bolus water drinking in older adults was superior to other non-pharmacological measures in decreasing systolic BP drop [24].

Postprandial Hypotension

Non-pharmacological interventions that have been shown to be useful for PPH include education, water drinking (to increase gastric distension), frequent smaller meals, modifying meal temperature, and postprandial exercise.

Patient Education

Education regarding the risk of falling 15–90 minutes after eating, remaining in a supine position following a meal, and giving hypotensive medications between meals is important.

Water Drinking

Avoiding preload reduction (diuretics or prolonged sitting) and maintaining adequate intravascular volume by drinking water have been shown to reduce postprandial drop in BP. In a small case-control study, drinking 400 ml of water before lunch elicited significant pressor effects by increasing systolic and diastolic pressure 13.9+/−4.7/5.2+/−2.2 mm Hg compared with blood pressure in the controls ($p < 0.005$). So drinking water before meal is recommended for older adults who experience postprandial hypotension [25]. In MSA patients with autonomic failure, drinking 350 ml of water before a meal reduced the magnitude of PPH by 21 mm Hg and 13 mm Hg, respectively, and that effect was sustained for 60 minutes [15]. Pressor response was postulated due to sympathetic activation via osmotic spinal afferents [15]. Water drinking has also been shown to be effective even within 5 minutes in attenuating postprandial fall in blood pressure [26].

Different Body Positions and Exercise

Different body positions alone do not adequately prevent PPH or attenuate drops in blood pressure for older adults with PPH [27]. After checking with ambulatory blood pressure readings, individual patients should remain recumbent for the period during which symptoms usually occur and through the nadir of BP drop.

Exercise has been studied as an intervention in few PPH studies. Two studies in elderly subjects showed walking exercise attenuated the postprandial hypotensive response to the meal, but this effect was only sustained for the duration of the exercise [28, 29]. In a small recent study in older adults with PPH, intermittent walking after ingestion of a glucose drink at a usual pace attenuated the drop in BP after the drink [30].

Types of Meals: Various types of meals account for the hypotensive response and are mediated by the products of their digestion and absorption. Simple carbohydrate like glucose showed greatest hypotensive response when compared to complex carbohydrate like starch, as this could be due to slower rate of small intestinal absorption [31–33]. Increase in sympathetic nervous system activity to counteract the effect of postprandial drop in blood pressure is a normal mechanism seen in individuals. In subjects with PPH, blunting of the normal increase in sympathetic activity and plasma norepinephrine levels after meals are seen [34–36].

Reducing the amount of rice (carbohydrates) intake per meal in a small study in nursing home residents showed that it helps prevent postprandial blood pressure

Table 7.3 Selected studies about non-pharmacological interventions

Study	Subjects	Interventions	Outcomes
El-Sayed (1996) Double blind placebo controlled trial [51]	20	Increased salt intake	Associated with increase in plasma volume and orthostatic intolerance
Claydon (2004) Case Series [52]	11	Salt supplementation of 100 mmol/day	Improved orthostatic intolerance
Deguchi (2007) Case Series [15]	5	Water drinking	Constant pressor effect on day 1 and day 7
Podoleanu (2006) Randomized cross-over study [23]	21	Compression bandage	Avoid BP drop and reduce symptoms
Fan (2011) Open RCT [18]	130	Elevation of the head of the bed	Was not associated with improvement in OH and symptoms
Van Dijk (2006) RCT [44]	223	Physical countermeasures	Reduction in vasovagal syncope burden with prodrome
Son (2015) A within-subjects repeated measures design [25]	39	Rice or carbohydrate intake in meals	Reducing the amount of rice intake per meal prevents postprandial blood pressure decrease
Newton JL (2018) Observational study [24]	25	Bolus water drinking, compression stockings, abdominal compression, physical counter maneuvers	Bolus water drinking is superior to other non-pharmacological measures

decrease in the older subjects. Small and frequent meals with decreased carbohydrate content were recommended to prevent postprandial hypotension and its complications in the older people [37] (Table 7.3).

Vloet et al. in their study used three different types of liquid carbohydrate [low (25 g), normal (65 g), and high (125 g)] by 12 older subjects with PPH. The study showed a significant maximum decrease in SBP in the low (28 ± 5 mm Hg) carbohydrate group compared to the normal (39 ± 7 mm Hg) and high (40 ± 5 mm Hg) carbohydrate groups. In addition, the duration of PPH was significantly shorter in the low carbohydrate group than in the other groups [38]. Cold food or drinks can slow down the gastric emptying, and temperature of the food can also play a role in PPH [39].

Vasovagal Syndrome

Patient Education

Patients should be reassured of the benign course of the condition, and counseling regarding recognition of prodromal symptoms is important [40].

Lifestyle Measures

Conservative lifestyle measures such as increasing fluid and salt intake and physical counter maneuvers (PCMs) are the first line of management in vasovagal syndrome (VVS). Overall fluid intake should be increased by up to 2–2.5 l per day, as well as salt intake provided there are no contraindications [41].

Physical Countermeasures

PCMs are risk free, low cost and should be used as first line management in VVS patients with prodromal symptoms [42].

Isometric exercise of the large muscles with leg crossing, tensing of leg, abdominal and buttock muscle, and arm tensing have been shown to induce a significant blood pressure increase during the prodromal phase of reflex syncope on tilt tests and helps avoid or delay transient loss of consciousness seen with VVS. PCMs were shown to be only effective in preventing VVS in patients who experience a prodrome [43, 44] (Table 7.3). However, a recent study (ISSUE 3) showed many patients had syncope recurrence despite PCMs, perhaps because of older age and lack of sufficiently long prodrome [45]. Tilt training or home orthostatic training, with prolonged periods in the upright position, is not currently recommended.

Carotid Sinus Hypersensitivity

Avoiding tight collar shirts and sudden head turning may be helpful. Patients are advised to take increased volumes of fluid (2 + litres/day) and, if safe, to increase salt consumption (> 3 g/day) in carotid sinus hypersensitivity subjects. The principle difficulty in management is the frequent coincidence of hypertension. This coincidence becomes even more important when drug therapy of recurrent syncope has to be considered. These interventions, which may offer benefit in supporting low blood pressure during symptoms, are likely to raise the blood pressure to unacceptable levels at all other times [46].

Exercise-Induced Hypotension

Non-pharmacological measures like performing exercise in sitting or supine positions will be helpful to avoid exercise-induced hypotension. Adequate fluid intake can improve blood pressure and post-exercise hypotension had been ameliorated in autonomic failure patients [47]. Avoiding food intake for several hours before exercise also helped to prevent postprandial hypotension and also diminished the hypotensive response to exercise [48]. Gentilcore et al. investigated the effects of high-intensity bicycle exercise on community-dwelling healthy elderly subjects following ingestion of a 300 ml glucose (75 gm) drink. Exercise exacerbated the hypotensive response of post-meal or post-glucose drink ingestion [49]

Nocturnal Hypotension

Nocturnal hypotension (extreme dippers) is closely associated with excessive morning BP surge and orthostatic hypertension [50]. Suggesting to raise slowly may help to prevent the orthostatic increase in BP, but no studies have been done so far to show that benefit.

Conclusions

Twenty-four hours ambulatory blood pressure measurement may assist in diagnosing overall low BP with different hypotensive syndromes. Potentially effective and relatively safe non-pharmacological measures should be considered as a therapeutic option in all hypotensive syndromes. Non-pharmacological measures should be the first line of management, but it is not always sufficient for subjects with symptomatic hypotensive syndromes. Treatment of hypotensive syndromes begins with patient's education by increasing the awareness of these hypotensive syndromes and symptoms. Lifestyle modifications such as increased fluid intake, avoiding large meals, and physical counter maneuvers have been shown to be effective as different non-pharmacological treatment options. However, data from randomized, controlled trials are limited. There is a need for more research with these non-pharmacological interventions in hypotensive syndromes.

References

1. Mills PB, Fung CK, Travlos A, et al. Nonpharmacologic management of orthostatic hypotension: a systematic review. Arch Phys Med Rehabil. 2015;96:366–75.
2. Rowell LB. Cardiovascular aspects of human thermoregulation. Circ Res. 1983;52:367–79.
3. Pathak A, Lapeyre-Mestre M, Montastruc JL, et al. Heat-related morbidity in patients with orthostatic hypotension and primary autonomic failure. Mov Disord. 2005;20:1213–9.
4. Petrofsky JS, Besonis C, Rivera D, et al. Impairment in orthostatic tolerance during heat exposure in individuals with type I and type II diabetes. Med Sci Monit. 2005;11:153–9.
5. Parsaik A, Allison TG, Singer W, et al. Deconditioning in patients with orthostatic intolerance. Neurology. 2012;79:1435–9.
6. Teri Harkell ADJ, Van Lieshout JJ, et al. Effects of leg muscle pumping and tensing on orthostatic arterial pressure: a study in normal subjects and patients with autonomic failure. Clin Sci. 1994;87:553–8.
7. Narkiewicz K, Cooley RL, Somers VK. Alcohol potentiates orthostatic hypotension: implications for alcohol-related syncope. Circulation. 2000;101:398–402.
8. Endo Y, Yamauchi K, Tsutsui Y, et al. Changes in blood pressure and muscle sympathetic nerve activity during water drinking in humans. Jpn J Physiol. 2002;52:421–7.
9. Rossi P, Andriesse GI, Oey PL, et al. Stomach distension increases efferent muscle sympathetic nerve activity and blood pressure in healthy humans. J Neurol Sci. 1998;161:148–55.
10. Lipp A, Tank J, Franke G, et al. Osmosensitive mechanisms contribute to the water-drinking-induced pressor response in humans. Neurology. 2005;65:905–7.
11. Jordan J, Shannon JR, Black BK, et al. The pressor response to water-drinking in humans: a sympathetic reflex? Circulation. 2000;101:504–9.

12. Mtinangi BL, Hainsworth R. Early effects of oral salt on plasma volume, orthostatic tolerance, and baroreceptor sensitivity in patients with syncope. Clin Auton Res. 1998;8:231–5.. (Rpt ref for salt).
13. Lahrmann H, Cortelli P, Hilz M, et al. EFNS guidelines on the diagnosis and management of orthostatic hypotension. Eur J Neurol. 2006;13:930–6.
14. Wieling W, Hainsworth R. Orthostatic tolerance: salt, water and the autonomic nervous system. Clin Auton Res. 2002;12:234–5.
15. Deguchi K, Ikeda K, Sasaki I, et al. Effects of daily water drinking on orthostatic and postprandial hypotension in patients with multiple system atrophy. J Neurol. 2007;254:735–40.
16. Waters WW, Platts SH, Mitchell BM, et al. Plasma volume restoration with salt tablets and water after bed rest prevents orthostatic hypotension and changes in supine hemodynamic and endocrine variables. Am J Physiol Heart Circ Physiol. 2005;288(2):H839–47.
17. Van Lieshout JJ, Ten Harkel DJ, Wieling W. Fludrocortisone and sleeping in the head up position limit the postural decrease in cardiac output in autonomic failure. Clin Auton Res. 2000;10:35–42.
18. Fan CW, Walsh C, Cunningham CJ. The effect of sleeping with the head of the bed elevated six inches on elderly patients with orthostatic hypotension and open randomized controlled trial. Age Ageing. 2011;40:187–92.
19. Maclean A, Allen E. Orthostatic hypotension and orthostatic tachycardia: Treatment with the head- up bed. J Am Med Ass. 1940;115:2162–7.
20. Bannister R, Sever P, Gross M. Cardiovascular reflexes and biochemical responses in progressive autonomic failure. Brain. 1977;100:327–44.
21. Denq JC, Opfer-Gehrking TL, Giuliani M, et al. Efficacy of compression of different capacitance beds in the amelioration of orthostatic hypotension. Clin Auton Res. 1997;7(6):321–6.
22. Smeenk HE, Koster MJ, Faaij RA, et al. Compression therapy in patients with orthostatic hypotension: a systematic review. Neth J Med. 2014;72(2):80–5.
23. Podoleanu C, Maggi R, Brignole M, et al. Lower limb and abdominal compression bandages prevent progressive orthostatic hypotension in elderly persons: a randomized single-blind controlled study. J Am Coll Cardiol. 2006;48(7):1425–32.
24. Newton JL, Frith J. The efficacy of nonpharmacologic intervention for orthostatic hypotension associated with aging. Neurology. 2018;91(7):e652–6.
25. Son JT, Lee E. Effect of water drinking on the postprandial fall of blood pressure in the elderly. J Korean Acad Fundam Nurs. 2010;17(3):304–13.
26. Shannon JR, Diedrich A, Biaggioni I, et al. Water drinking as a treatment for orthostatic syndromes. Am J Med. 2002;112:355–60.
27. Tae Son J, Lee E. Comparison of postprandial blood pressure reduction in the elderly by different body position. Geriatr Nurs. 2013;34:282–8.
28. Jonsson PV, Lipsitz LA, Kelley M, et al. Hypotensive responses to common daily activities in institutionalized elderly. A potential risk for recurrent falls. Arch Intern Med. 1990;150:1518–24.
29. Oberman AS, Harada RK, Gagnon MM, et al. Effects of postprandial walking exercise on meal-related hypotension in frail elderly patients. Am J Cardiol. 1999;84:1130–2.
30. Nair S, Visvanathan R, Gentilcore D. Intermittent walking: a potential treatment for older people with postprandial hypotension. J Am Med Dir Assoc. 2015;16:160–4.
31. Potter JF, Heseltine D, Hartley G, et al. Effects of meal composition on the postprandial blood pressure, catecholamine and insulin changes in elderly subjects. Clin Sci (Lond). 1989;77:265–72.
32. Heseltine D, Dakkak M, Macdonald IA, et al. Effects of carbohydrate type on postprandial blood pressure, neuroendocrine and gastrointestinal hormone changes in the elderly. Clin Auton Res. 1991;1:219–24.
33. Visvanathan R, Horowitz M, Chapman I. The hypotensive response to oral fat is comparable but slower compared with carbohydrate in healthy elderly subjects. Br J Nutr. 2006;95:340–5.
34. Masuda Y, Kawamura A. Role of the autonomic nervous system in postprandial hypotension in elderly persons. J Cardiovasc Pharmacol. 2003;42:S23–6.

35. Fagius J, Ellerfelt K, Lithell H, et al. Increase in muscle nerve sympathetic activity after glucose intake is blunted in the elderly. Clin Auton Res. 1996;6:195–203.
36. Mitro P, Feterik K, Lenártová M, et al. Humoral mechanisms in the pathogenesis of postprandial hypotension in patients with essential hypertension. Wien Klin Wochenschr. 2001;113:424–32.
37. Tae Son J, Lee E. Effects of the amount of rice in meals on postprandial blood pressure in older people with postprandial hypotension: a within-subjects design. J Clin Nurs. 2015;24:2277–85.
38. Vloet LC, Mehagnoul-Schipper DJ, Hoefnagels WH, et al. The influence of low-, normal-, and high-carbohydrate meals on blood pressure in elderly patients with postprandial hypotension. J Gerontol A Biol Sci Med Sci. 2001;56:M744–8.
39. Sun WM, Houghton LA, Read NW, et al. Effect of meal temperature on gastric emptying of liquids in man. Gut. 1988;29:302–5.
40. Parry SW, Kenny RA. The management of vasovagal syncope. Q J Med. 1999;92:697–705.
41. Wieling W, Colman N, Krediet CT, Freeman R. Nonpharmacological treatment of reflex syncope. Clin Auton Res. 2004;14(Suppl 1):62–70.
42. Sheldon RS, Grubb BP, Olshansky B, et al. 2015 heart rhythm society expert consensus statement on the diagnosis and treatment of postural tachycardia syndrome, inappropriate sinus tachycardia, and vasovagal syncope. Heart Rhythm. 2015;12:e41–63.
43. Krediet CT, van Dijk N, LinzerMvanLieshout JJ, et al. Management of vasovagal syncope: controlling or aborting faints by leg crossing and muscle tensing. Circulation. 2002;106:1684–9.
44. van Dijk N, Quartieri F, Blanc JJ, et al. Effectiveness of physical counterpressure maneuvers in preventing vasovagal syncope: the physical CounterpressureManoeuvres trial (PC-trial). J Am Coll Cardiol. 2006;48:1652–7.
45. Tomaino M, Romeo C, Vitale E, et al. Physical counter-pressure manoeuvres in preventing syncopal recurrence in patients older than 40 years with recurrent neurally mediated syncope: a controlled study from the Third International Study on Syncope of Uncertain Etiology (ISSUE-3) dagger. Europace. 2014;16:1515–20.
46. Romme JJ, Reitsma JB, Black CN, et al. Drugs and pacemakers for vasovagal, carotid sinus and situational syncope. Cochrane Database Syst Rev. 2011;(10):CD004194.
47. Humm AM, Mason LM, Mathias CJ. Effects of water drinking on cardiovascular responses to supine exercise and on orthostatic hypotension after exercise in pure autonomic failure. J Neurol Neurosurg Psychiatry. 2008;79:1160–4.
48. Puvi-Rajasingham S, Smith GD, Akinola A, et al. Hypotensive and regional haemodynamic effects of exercise, fasted and after food, in human sympathetic denervation. Clin Sci (Lond). 1998;94:49–55.
49. Gentilcore D, Nair NS, Kuo P, et al. Effects of aerobic exercise on gastric emptying of, and the glycemic and cardiovascular responses to oral glucose in healthy older subjects. Neurogastroenterol Motil. 2008;20:83.
50. Kario K, Eguchi K, Nakagawa Y, et al. Relationship between extreme dippers and orthostatic hypertension in elderly hypertensive patients. Hypertension. 1998;31:77–82.
51. El-Sayed H, Hainsworth R. Salt supplement increases plasma volume and orthostatic tolerance in patients with unexplained syncope. Heart. 1996;75:134–40.
52. Claydon VE, Hainsworth R. Salt supplementation improves orthostatic cerebral and peripheral vascular control in patients with syncope. Hypertension. 2004;43:809–13.

Update on Pharmacological Management of Hypotensive Syndromes in the Elderly

8

Kannayiram Alagiakrishnan and Darren Mah

Introduction

Hypotensive syndromes can be caused by autonomic failure and may occur secondary to a disease or its treatment. Autonomic failure can lead to many of the hypotensive syndromes, including orthostatic hypotension (OH), post-prandial hypotension (PPH), post-exercise hypotension (PEH), vasovagal syndrome (VVS) and carotid sinus syndrome (CSS). Overtreatment of hypertension, especially in the frail elderly, can also result in OH and PPH [1].

Addressing Offending Medications: A Critical First Step in the Medical Management of Hypotensive Syndromes

Many medications, including diuretics, alpha blockers, vasodilators, tricyclic antidepressants, certain antipsychotics and medications used for Parkinson's disease (PD) like levodopa and dopamine agonists, can cause OH (Table 8.1). Addressing drug-induced hypotension is an important initial step, as reducing medication doses and/or changing medications entirely may lead to significant improvement [2]. In a study on deprescribing medications in a syncope clinic, 35% of persons with a principal diagnosis of orthostatic hypotension and for whom medications were stopped experienced symptom improvement [3].

K. Alagiakrishnan (✉)
Division of Geriatric Medicine, University of Alberta, Edmonton, AB, Canada

D. Mah
University of Alberta, Edmonton, AB, Canada

© Springer Nature Switzerland AG 2020
K. Alagiakrishnan, M. Banach (eds.), *Hypotensive Syndromes in Geriatric Patients*, https://doi.org/10.1007/978-3-030-30332-7_8

Table 8.1 Important medications that induce hypotension

Antihypertensive agents
Diuretics
Alpha blockers
Beta blockers without intrinsic sympathomimetic activity
Combined alpha and beta blockers
Calcium channel blockers – long acting and dihydropyridine
Parkinsonian medications
Dopaminergic agonists
Levodopa
Selegiline
Psychotropic medications
Antipsychotics
Tricyclic antidepressants
Monoamine oxidase inhibitors
Trazodone

Antihypertensive Medications

Thiazide, loop and potassium-sparing diuretics reduce preload and can lead to OH [4]. In epidemiologic studies of patients with Parkinson's disease, diuretics more than quintupled the risk of OH [5]. Yoshimura et al. in a survey of the FDA Adverse Events Reporting System database found an increased risk of OH with different alpha blockers, with odds ratios for doxasozin, tamsulosin, alfuzosin and terazosin of 2.66, 3.31, 4.21 and 6.13, respectively [6]. Calcium channel blockers, through natriuresis and vasodilation, may also lead to the development of OH [7, 8].

Additionally, non-dihydropyridine calcium channel blockers may cause OH through negative effects on cardiac contractility and conduction, preventing compensatory increases in heart rate upon standing [9]. Both nifedipine and the nitroglycerine patch have been shown to significantly decrease systolic blood pressure. However, at doses that yielded the same systolic blood pressure drop, nifedipine led to worse morning OH, likely due to nocturnal natriuresis [10]. Slavachevsky et al. found enalapril led to fewer OH episodes compared to long-acting nifedipine [11]. Centrally acting alpha-2 agonists like clonidine, a central sympatholytic agent, and beta blockers with combined alpha blocker activity such as labetalol can also cause OH. The reported prevalence of OH with labetalol was 1.4% [12]. In addition to nitrates and calcium channel blockers, vasodilators such as phosphodiesterase E5 inhibitors like sildenafil, vardenafil and tadalafil can also cause OH.

Among older adults with adequate hypertensive control, the prevalence of OH is low [13]. However, an increased occurrence of PPH is seen among individuals with systolic hypertension [14, 15]. For individuals with hypertension who experience OH, management should aim for adequate treatment of hypertension and avoidance of antihypertensive medications that cause OH. Adequate treatment of hypertension and avoidance of diuretics and nitrates can help to reduce postprandial blood pressure drop [16].

Parkinsonian Medications

OH is also seen with anti-Parkinson's medications like levodopa [17] and dopamine agonists [18]. In PD, OH has been shown to be a well-recognized adverse effect of all available dopamine agonists, including bromocriptine, pergolide, and newer agents such as pramipexole and ropinirole [19, 20]. A small study showed that levodopa/benserazide therapy (50 mg/12.5 mg twice daily) did not increase the incidence of PH or PPH in older adults with Parkinson's disease; however, when higher-dose therapy is indicated in elderly patients, careful orthostatic and postprandial BP monitoring may be advisable because hypotensive side effects may then become more pronounced [21]. Selegiline has also been shown to induce OH [22].

Psychotropic Medications

Numerous drugs used to treat psychiatric disorders also may contribute to OH. Both typical and atypical antipsychotic drugs, regardless of potency, have shown to increase rates of OH, especially those with significant alpha-1 antagonism such as clozapine and quetiapine [23]. Tricyclic antidepressants, despite their known anticholinergic properties, can cause OH and therefore may increase fall risk. The tricyclic antidepressants with the greatest known risk for the development of OH are amitriptyline, imipramine and doxepin. Other medications such as monoamine oxidase inhibitors and trazodone are commonly implicated in the development of OH [24].

Existing and Emerging Therapies for Hypotensive Syndromes

Existing Therapies

To date, available therapy for hypotensive syndromes is lacking in efficacy and evidence. Most antihypotensive medications have been assessed only in small trials. Additionally, these studies have often looked only at vital signs instead of symptomatic control and/or functional improvement. Further research will be important to determine long-term effects and side effects of these medications.

Current medications use different mechanisms to try to combat hypotensive syndromes. Midodrine, pyridostigmine and yohimbine exert their effects by increasing peripheral resistance. Fludrocortisone sensitizes alpha-adrenoreceptors and increases sodium and water resorption. In clinical practice, to combat hypotensive syndromes, these medications are titrated to their highest tolerable dose and/or given in conjunction with other blood pressure increasing drugs. However, these medications are slightly limited in their clinical use as they tend to severely increase blood pressure, especially when supine [25] (Table 8.2).

Table 8.2 Medications used in different hypotensive syndromes

Medications	OH	PPH	VVS	CSS	PEH
Fludrocortisone	Yes	No	Yes	No	No
Midodrine	Yes	Yes	Yes	Yes	Yes
Droxidopa	Yes	Yes	No	No	No
Octreotide	Yes	Yes	No	No	No
Caffeine	Yes	Yes	No	No	No
Salt tablets	Yes	No	Yes	No	No
Pyridostigmine	Yes	No	No	No	No
Atomoxetine	Yes	No	No	No	No
SSRI	No	No	Yes	Yes	No
Beta blockers	No	No	Yes	Yes	No

Adapted from Alagiakrishnan [25]

OH orthostatic hypotension, *PPH* postprandial hypotension, *VVS* vasovagal syndrome, *CSS* carotid sinus syndrome, *PEH* post-exercise hypotension

Emerging Therapies

Droxidopa: Droxidopa is a synthetic norepinephrine prodrug that is converted into norepinephrine in both central nervous system and peripheral tissues, causing peripheral vasoconstriction [26]. Its duration of action ranges from 6 to 8 hours, depending on if the patient remains standing or supine. It can be considered as an additional therapy for OH if medical management with other antihypotensive drugs has failed [27]. Phase 3 studies have demonstrated significant symptom improvement of OH and improvement in activities of daily living with droxidopa. It has been shown to decrease common symptoms such as dizziness, lightheadedness, weakness and fatigue, and has also been associated with a reduced number of falls [28, 29]. Like other medications used to treat OH, droxidopa should not be taken within 5 hours of going to sleep in order to decrease the risk of supine hypertension [30]. Data on the long-term effectiveness of droxidopa is lacking.

Atomoxetine: Atomoxetine is a noradrenaline reuptake inhibitor which acts akin to a vasopressor. In a small clinical trial, atomoxetine increased standing blood pressure more when compared to midodrine. Even small doses of atomoxetine have shown a significant increase in blood pressure [31]. Atomoxetine may be a reasonable alternative when other medications fail to improve hypotensive symptoms. Long term studies showing effect are lacking [32, 33].

Mirabegron: Mirabegron is a beta-3 adrenergic receptor agonist primarily used to treat overactive bladder (OAB). Given its stimulatory effects on the cardiovascular system, it has been considered for the treatment of OH. Anecdotally, it has been used off-label in people with comorbid OAB and OH as a means of avoiding the vasodepressor effects of anticholinergic alternatives. However, the United Kingdom's Medicines and Healthcare Products Regulatory Agency has issued a drug safety update concerning the risk of severe hypertension with mirabegron [34].

Further clinical trials are required before considering this agent for use in clinical practice. Currently the evidence points out that more research is needed and suggests the risks may outweigh the benefits seen with this medication.

Steps to Prevent Supine Hypertension and Its Sequelae Due to the Treatment of Hypotensive Syndromes

Supine hypertension is a common finding in autonomic failure [35]. Neurodegenerative disorders such as Parkinson's disease, multiple system atrophy, dementia with Lewy bodies and peripheral neuropathies cause neurogenic orthostatic hypotension (nOH) and may also be associated with supine hypertension. Mild supine hypertension (systolic blood pressure up to 160 mmHg) should be monitored closely, especially if the symptoms of OH have improved. However, it is recommended to treat severe supine hypertension (>180/110 mmHg) using short-acting antihypertensive agents at nighttime, as patients are typically supine for an extended period of time [36].

Many medications used to treat hypotensive syndromes in autonomic insufficiency can also cause supine hypertension, especially fludrocortisone. In such a case, changing to a short-acting pressor agent (e.g. midodrine, droxidopa, etc.) may sometimes help. Pyridostigmine may also reduce postural blood pressure drop without causing supine hypertension. The addition of short-acting hypertensives is another strategy that can be tried but must but individually tailored. Different therapeutic steps have been suggested to treat supine hypertension without inducing OH, but no single treatment approach has been studied in detail.

Raising the head of the bed 10–20 degrees above parallel may protect the brain from the effects of supine hypertension [25]. Identifying sympathetic denervation can help guide treatment for patients with nOH and supine hypertension. In patient with intact sympathetic function, using pyridostigmine improves symptoms of OH through increasing sympathetic activity, but if supine hypertension develops, a blood pressure medication which reduces sympathetic tone such as clonidine can be used. In patients with minimal residual activity, direct vasoconstrictors like midodrine and fludrocortisone can help to improve OH, and if these patients develop supine hypertension, direct vasodilators (i.e., nitroglycerine patch, calcium channel blockers) may ameliorate the problem [37, 38].

Conclusions

Hypotensive syndromes are common conditions seen in the elderly. The first step in the pharmacological management of these syndromes is stopping, changing or decreasing the dose of offending medication(s). Among the existing therapies, fludrocortisone, midodrine and pyridostigmine are commonly used. Emerging treatments that can be useful include droxidopa and atomoxetine. Different therapeutic approaches can be used to treat hypertension associated with hypotensive syndromes and their treatment, although these require longer-term studies in assessing their efficacy.

References

1. Morley JE. Hypertension—is it overtreated in the elderly. J Am Med Dir Assoc. 2010;11:147–52.
2. Poon IO, Braun U. High prevalence of orthostatic hypotension and its correlation with potentially causative medications among elderly veterans. J Clin Pharm Ther. 2005;30(2):173–8.
3. Alsop K, MacMohan M. Withdrawing cardiovascular medications at a syncope clinic. Postgrad Med J. 2001;77:403–5.
4. Arnold AC, Shibao C. Current concepts in orthostatic hypotension management. Curr Hypertens Rep. 2013;15(4):304–12.
5. Perez-Lloret S, Rey MV, Fabre N, et al. Factors related to orthostatic hypotension in Parkinson's disease. Parkinsonism Relat Disord. 2012;18(5):501–5.
6. Yoshimura K, Kadoyama K, Sakaeda T, et al. A survey of the FAERS database concerning the adverse event profiles of alpha1-adrenoreceptor blockers for lower urinary tract symptoms. Int J Med Sci. 2013;10(7):864–9.
7. Hajjar I. Postural blood pressure changes and orthostatic hypotension in the elderly patient: impact of antihypertensive medications. Drugs Aging. 2005;22:55–68.
8. Masuo K, Mikami H, Ogihara T, et al. Changes in frequency of orthostatic hypotension in elderly hypertensive patients under medications. Am J Hypertens. 1996;9:263–8.
9. Milazzo V, Di Stefano C, Servo S, et al. Drugs and orthostatic hypotension: evidence from literature. J Hypertens. 2012;1(2):1–8.
10. Jordan J, Shannon JR, Pohar B, et al. Contrasting effects of vasodilators on blood pressure and sodium balance in the hypertension of autonomic failure. J Am Soc Nephrol. 1999;10:35–42.
11. Slavachevsky I, Rachmani R, Levi Z, et al. Effect of enalapril on orthostatic hypotension in older hypertensive patients. J Am Geriatr Soc. 2000;48(7):807–10.
12. Pearce CJ, Wallin JD. Labetalol and other agents that block alpha and beta- adrenergic receptors. Cleve Clin J Med. 1994;61(1):59–69.
13. Saez T, Suarez C, Sierra MJ, et al. Orthostatic hypotension in the aged and its association with antihypertensive treatment. Med Clin (Barc). 2000;114:525–9.
14. Mitro P, Feterik K, Cverckova A, et al. Occurrence and relevance of postprandial hypotension in patients with essential hypertension. Wien Klin Wochenschr. 1999;111:320–5.
15. Grodzicki T, Rajzer M, Fagard R, et al. Ambulatory blood pressure monitoring and postprandial hypotension in elderly patients with isolated systolic hypertension. J Hum Hypertens. 1998;12:161–5.
16. Alagiakrishnan K. Postural and postprandial hypotension: approach to management. Geriatr Aging. 2007;10(5):298–304.
17. McDowell FH, Lee JE. Levodopa, Parkinson's disease, and hypotension. Ann Intern Med. 1970;72:751–2.
18. Kujawa K, Leurgans S, Raman R, et al. Acute orthostatic hypotension when starting dopamine agonists in Parkinson's disease. Arch Neurol. 2000;57:1461–3.
19. Dooley M, Markham A. Pramipexole: a review of its use in the management of early and advanced Parkinson's disease. Drugs Aging. 1998;12:495–514.
20. Johns DW, Ayers CR, Carey RM. The dopamine agonist bromocriptine induces hypotension by venous and arteriolar dilation. J Cardiovasc Pharmacol. 1984;6:582–7.
21. Mehagnoul-Schipper DJ, Boerman RH, Hoefnagels WHL, et al. Effects of levodopa on orthostatic and postprandial hypotension in elderly parkinsonian patients. J Gerontol A Biol Sci Med Sci. 2001;56:M749–55.

22. Churchyard A, Mathias CJ, Lees AJ. Selegiline-induced postural hypotension in Parkinson's disease: a longitudinal study on the effects of drug withdrawal. Mov Disord. 1999;14(2):246–51.
23. Gugger JJ. Antipsychotic pharmacotherapy and orthostatic hypotension: identification and management. CNS Drugs. 2011;25(8):659–71.
24. American Psychiatric Association practice guidelines. American Psychiatric Association website. http://www.psychiatry-online.org/guidelines. Accessed 19 Nov 2018.
25. Alagiakrishnan K. Current pharmacological management of hypotensive syndromes in the elderly. Drugs Aging. 2015;32:337–48.
26. Biaggioni I, Hewitt AL, Rowse GJ, et al. Integrated analysis of droxidopa trials for neurogenic orthostatic hypotension. BMC Neurol. 2017;17:90.
27. Keating GM. Droxidopa: a review of its use in symptomatic neurogenic orthostatic hypotension. Drugs. 2015;75(2):197–206.
28. Kaufmann H, Freeman R, Biaggioni I, et al. Droxidopa for neurogenic orthostatic hypotension: a randomized, placebo-controlled, phase 3 trial. Neurology. 2014;83(4):328–35.
29. Hauser RA, Isaacson S, Lisk JP, et al. Droxidopa for the short-term treatment of symptomatic neurogenic orthostatic hypotension in Parkinson's disease (nOH306B). Mov Disord. 2015;30(5):646–54.
30. Hauser RA, Hewitt LA, Isaacson S. Droxidopa in patients with neurogenic orthostatic hypotension associated with Parkinson's disease (NOH306A). J Park Dis. 2014;4(1):57–65.
31. Ramirez CE, Okamoto LE, Arnold AC, et al. Efficacy of atomoxetine versus midodrine for the treatment of orthostatic hypotension in autonomic failure. Hypertension. 2014;64:1235–40.
32. Hale GM, Brenner M. Atomoxetine for orthostatic hypotension in an elderly patient over 10 weeks: a case report. Pharmacology. 2015;35:e141–8.
33. Kasi PM, Mounzer R, Gleeson GH. Cardiovascular side effects of atomoxetine and its interactions with inhibitors of the cytochrome p450 system. Case Rep Med. 2011;2011:1–3.
34. MHRA. 2015. Accessed at gov.uk at http://www.webcitation.org/6dLqnZooZ. 27 Nov 2015, date last accessed.
35. Jordan J, Biaggioni I. Diagnosis and treatment of supine hypertension in autonomic failure patients with orthostatic hypotension. J Clin Hypertens (Greenwich). 2002;4(2):139–45.
36. Gibbons CH, Schmidt P, Biaggioni I, et al. The recommendations of a consensus panel for the screening, diagnosis, and treatment of neurogenic orthostatic hypotension and associated supine hypertension. J Neurol. 2017;264(8):1567–82.
37. Shannon JR, Jordan J, Diedrich A, et al. Sympathetically mediated hypertension in autonomic failure. Circulation. 2000;101:2710–5.
38. Baker J, Kimpinski K. Management of supine hypertension complicating neurogenic orthostatic hypotension. CNS Drugs. 2017;31(8):653–63.

Challenges with the Diagnosis and Management of Hypotensive Syndromes in the Elderly

Kannayiram Alagiakrishnan

Introduction

Hemodynamic homeostasis become less effective with aging and is associated with a decreased ability to regulate blood pressure. Hypotensive syndromes are low blood pressure (BP) conditions seen in the supine or with position changes in older adults. It is defined as lower BP than usual in lying and standing positions, with head turning and after meals. Prevalence of these conditions varies with age, different co-morbid conditions, and different living situations. 24-hour ambulatory blood pressure recording offers the potential to capture different hypotensive events. In this chapter, we will discuss about the challenges with the diagnosis and management of these hypotensive syndromes.

Challenges with Diagnosis

Orthostatic Hypotension

Issues with Consensus Definition
In 1996, the Consensus Committee of the American Autonomic Society and the American Academy of Neurology clinically defined orthostatic hypotension (OH) as "a reduction of systolic blood pressure of at least 20 mmHg or diastolic blood pressure of at least 10 mmHg within 3 minutes of standing" from a supine position [1]. This was based on clinical judgment, as epidemiologic data were not available at the time. In each of these elements, there exist issues that argue for modification of the presently accepted consensus criteria of OH. Consensus definition is appropriate for screening and standardization in clinical research, but it has

K. Alagiakrishnan (✉)
Division of Geriatric Medicine, University of Alberta, Edmonton, AB, Canada

© Springer Nature Switzerland AG 2020
K. Alagiakrishnan, M. Banach (eds.), *Hypotensive Syndromes in Geriatric Patients*, https://doi.org/10.1007/978-3-030-30332-7_9

limitations in the clinical care of the elderly patient with orthostatic symptoms. Optimal time duration of orthostatic challenge for the diagnosis of orthostatic hypotension is probably longer than the 3 min set in the consensus definition. It does not include patients who develop OH after longer periods of standing (delayed OH) [2].

1. Postural symptoms without meeting the OH criteria: It does not take into account those who have postural symptoms at drop in blood pressure of <20/10 mm Hg. Study by Ensrud et al. in their prospective cohort study showed postural dizziness was more strongly associated than postural hypotension with history of falling, syncope, and impaired functional status [3]. A majority of patients with severe orthostatic hypotension are asymptomatic or have atypical complaints. Atypical symptoms, such as lower extremity discomfort, backache, and headache, or even complete absence of symptoms occur in over half of our patients [4].

2. Types of OH

   Classical OH: It is a sustained reduction in systolic BP of 20 mm Hg or diastolic BP of 10 mm Hg within 3 minutes of standing or head-up tilt.

   Initial OH: Initial OH is defined as a transient SBP decrease of >40 mm Hg and/or diastolic BP decrease >20 mm Hg within 30 seconds of standing. The mechanism involves a mismatch between sudden decrease in venous return and neurally mediated compensatory vasoconstriction. Continuous BP monitoring helps to diagnose initial OH [5].

   OH in hypertensive subjects: OH was defined differently in patients with hypertension. Federowski et al. in their study found that the previous consensus criteria for the diagnosis of orthostatic hypotension needs modification. With normotensive subjects, the definition of SBP drop of >20 mm of Hg and DBP drop of >10 mm of Hg is reasonable. However in hypertension subjects (SBP >160 mm of Hg), systolic blood pressure drop of 30 mm of Hg instead of the standard 20 mm of Hg and in subjects whose SBP <115 mm of Hg, the systolic cutoff should be 15 mm of Hg [6, 7].

   Delayed OH: It is a reduction in orthostatic BP that occurs after 3 min of standing or head-up tilt. Both delayed OH and vasovagal syncope can cause blood pressure falls and can result in syncope; however, these are very different disorders. In patients with vasovagal syncope, tilt table testing will reveal a sudden, rapid fall in blood pressure, often with an associated relative bradycardia and prodromal symptoms that could include diaphoresis, nausea, and a feeling of warmth. This is in contrast to delayed OH, where there is typically no decrease in heart rate [8].

   Transient OH: It is defined as a drop in BP meeting OH criteria in the standing position at 1 or 3 or 6 min.

   Persistent OH: It is defined as a drop in BP at all the three time points 1, 3 and 6 min [9, 10].

   Subclinical OH: It is defined as a systolic drop of <20 mm Hg or diastolic drop of <10 mm of Hg with orthostatic hypotension symptoms [11, 12].

Delayed OH

Delayed OH is defined as a SBP drop of 20 mm of Hg or more, or DBP drop of 10 mm Hg or more after 3 minutes of upright posture by standing or upright tilt [2, 13]. Gibbons et al. in their observational study of 108 subjects with OH by tilt table testing found 46% had classic OH (within 3 minutes) and 54% had delayed OH (after 3 minutes). Out of the subjects with delayed OH, 15% had between 3 and 10 minutes, 39% had after 10 minutes [14]. In a pilot study from India, Grace Roy et al. showed delayed OH occurred in 42% of subjects and the incidence of delayed OH after 10 minutes was seen in 66% of subjects [15]. The study by Podoleanu et al. reported average time to symptom onset in delayed OH subjects was about 8.6 minutes [16]. A small study in adult women with age ranging between 30 and 65 years showed the prevalence of delayed OH in 25% of subjects [17]. All the symptoms seen with classical OH such as visual blurring due to retinal or occipital ischemia, gait unsteadiness, falls, coat hanger headache and neck pain on prolonged standing due to ischemia of the trapezius and neck muscles, fatigue on exertion, and orthostatic dyspnea due to impaired coronary circulation perfusion in spite of normal arteries [18, 19]. A 10-year follow-up study of delayed OH showed 54% develop also classical OH and with a substantial increase of neurodegenerative diseases like α-synucleinopathies as well as mortality [20].

Mechanisms of Delayed OH

Possible mechanisms for delayed OH could be due to increased microvascular filtration and peripheral venous swelling as well as the gradual failure of the humoral and neuromuscular mechanisms that counteract the gravitational redistribution of fluid [14]. With standing there is an increase in gravity related hydrostatic pressure with increased pooling which leads to microvascular filtration into surrounding tissues. In order to counter these effects, the increase in muscle sympathetic activity results in vessel constriction and increase in muscle tone which returns venous and lymphatic fluid from the dependant tissues back to the circulatory system [21–25]. Stimulation of cutaneous receptors in the foot causes calf muscle pump stimulation which can improve lymphatic return and can limit orthostatic blood pressure drop [26].

Diagnostic Dilemma of Delayed OH with VVS

The absence of bradycardia or pauses usually differentiates delayed OH from reflex syncope (VVS), although mixed forms are often encountered in clinical practice [27]. Head-up tilt testing can also be used for diagnosing delayed OH [28]. Tilt table records blood pressure and pulse after a 70 degree tilt using a motorized table. You can have the tilt up to 20 minutes. It helps to diagnose delayed OH. Some people argue it does not simulate real-life situation.

3. Validity of Testing (Reproducibility and Accuracy)
    (a) Even though day-to-day reproducibility of the diagnosis of OH, based on conventional criteria, were found to be poor [29]. In the study by Ward et al., the drop in blood pressure was more likely to be reproducible in the morning

than in the afternoon, which suggests evaluations be made in the morning [30]. Feasibility of detecting OH has been better by checking OH every day morning [31]. In hospital settings, postural blood pressure readings can be measured in the morning. Home monitoring is possible only if the patient is compliant.

(b) Problems with the diagnosis of OH are seen with BP measurement techniques (accuracy) which plays a role in the validity of testing. The skills necessary to measure OH are discussed below.

Bladder Size

Use a standard bladder (12–13 cm long and 35 cm wide) but have a larger and a smaller bladder available for obese and thin arms. The bladder dimensions are very important in relation to the arm circumference. If the bladder is too long there may be blood pressure underestimation and if it is short, blood pressure may be overestimated called "cuff hypertension" [32].

Posture

Blood pressure is affected by posture and normally there should be a slight increase from the lying to the sitting or standing position. Sources of error in the measurement technique become especially important in the sitting and standing positions, when the arm is likely to be dependent by the subject's side. Significant error in posture can be avoided if the arm is supported at the heart level.

Arm Support

If the arm is extended and left unsupported diastolic blood pressure may raise by as much as 10%. So it is essential that the health professional checking the blood pressure should hold the subject's arm at the elbow during blood pressure measurement. Even in the supine position an error of 5 mm Hg for diastolic pressure may occur if the arm is not supported at the heart level [33].

Arm Position

The level of the heart as denoted by the midsternal level and the arm must be horizontal at that level. If the arm is above heart level, it can underestimate systolic and diastolic blood pressures, and if it is below heart level, it can cause overestimation of these readings. This error can be as great as 10 mm Hg for systolic and diastolic pressures [33].

Pulse Checking

The pulse should also be checked with the blood pressure measurement in lying and standing position. If the pulse rate response increase is less than 15/min with the drop in the blood pressure it could be due to autonomic insufficiency. If pulse rate is more than 15/min, it could be due to volume loss or "POTS" (positional orthostatic tachycardia syndrome). POTS can be associated with considerable disability [34].

Another methodological question that needs to be addressed is the number of measurements required in order to establish a clinical diagnosis of orthostatic hypotension [35].

4. Sit to Stand Orthostatic Stress

   Sitting and standing blood pressure measurements are not accurate for diagnosing orthostatic hypotension [36]. Orthostatic stress tests (sit to stand-not enough stress) and also passive tilt with head-up/tilt table test do not stimulate real-life situation.

5. OH Using Central and Peripheral BP

   In the study by Tabara et al. when carotid and brachial blood pressure were measured simultaneously using cuff-oscillometric and tonometric methods, the orthostatic decline in blood pressure was more prominent in the carotid artery and orthostatic symptoms were better reflected by central blood pressure [37], whereas the study by Alagiakrishnan K et al. showed prevalence of OH was similar between PBP and CBP. This study showed the association of OH with arterial wall stiffness markers (augmentation pressure (AP) and augmentation index (AI)), as the alteration of the reflection pressure wave due to arterial wall stiffness could be one of the underlying mechanisms of OH in the central artery [9].

Postprandial Hypotension

1. Absence of a Standardized Consensus Definition

   Postprandial hypotension (PPH) lacks a standard definition on the magnitude of drop (systolic 20 mm or 30 mm drop) even though both the measurements as mentioned above have been used in different studies. The definition used by Lipsitz LA is a systolic BP drop of 20 mm of Hg [38]. However in a study on hypertensive subjects, a definition of SBP drop of 30 mm of Hg drop has been used [7]. But in a study by Narendar et al. showed that with a definition of PPH as >30 mm Hg systolic drop, will miss PPH in one of three patients when the blood pressure was measured every 10 minutes for 1 hour. In this study with the definition of PPH as >30 mm Hg drop, the presence of postprandial complaints was not associated with the existence of PPH [39]. PPH-related symptoms were significantly associated with a definition of SBP fall of greater than 20 mm of Hg (P < 0.001), rather than a SBP fall of >30 mm Hg (not significant) [39]. But there is no consensus on the test conditions that should be used to diagnose PPH. Standardized test meals were used in most of the studies.

2. Timing of the Postprandial Drop in Blood Pressure Is Variable

   The time interval for these measurements varied from 60 minutes to 120 minutes. Some studies used mercury sphygmomanometer, others had used Dinamap, Spacelab or 24-hour ambulatory blood pressure monitoring (ABPM) [40–43]. Postprandial drop in blood pressure can occur at different times in patients. In some studies drop has occurred as early as 15 minutes and reaches the lowest level around 60 minutes in 70% of subjects [7]. Patients are likely experience some discomfort if the frequency of measurements is too frequent. Some studies used continuous blood pressure measurements using 24-hour ambulatory blood pressure or Spacelabs.

3. Additive Effect of Postural Hypotension

Postprandial and postural hypotension can occur together. In this study by Imai et al., effects of meal ingestion and active standing on blood pressure were not additive [44]. But in a controlled paired comparison design study in elderly subjects, increased symptomatic hypotension was observed after meal ingestion and head-up tilt table testing. The effect of meal ingestion on hypotension and head-up tilt table testing were additive in this study [45].

4. Reproducibility of PPH

In a small study which included 42 women and 8 males, with a mean age of 83 ± 8 years, when the morning test results were compared on two consecutive days, the intraindividual reproducibility of PPH was good (kappa coefficient = 0.6) [46].

5. No Patient Friendly, Practical and Adequate Way of Monitoring in the Community

In a study of hypertensive subjects, the value of home blood pressure monitoring (HBPM) as a screening test for measuring asymptomatic postprandial hypotension was assessed by measuring BP before and after lunches on three consecutive days [47]. In a cross-sectional French study by Abbas et al., a new simplified diagnostic method for PPH in older people has been introduced. Systolic BP decrease of at least 10 mm Hg between BP measures before the meal and 75 minutes after the end of the meal as the new definition of PPH. This new method had a sensitivity of 82% and a specificity of 91% and may be suitable and efficient for older adults [48] (Table 9.1).

Table 9.1 Challenges with the diagnosis of hypotensive syndromes

1. OH
(a) Symptomatic OH without meeting the criteria.
(b) Different types of OH including delayed OH.
(c) Reproducibility is poor.
(d) Validity (accuracy) of testing.
(e) Sit to stand testing (not enough of orthostatic stress).
2. PPH
(a) Lacks a standard definition.
(b) No patient friendly, practical way of measurement in the community.
3. CSS
Different diagnostic criteria.
4. VVS:
(a) Different tilt table testing protocols.
(b) Reproducibility is limited.
5. PEH
Different diagnostic criteria.
6. Nocturnal hypotension
Diagnosed only by doing 24-hour ambulatory BP monitoring.

Carotid Sinus Syndrome

Carotid sinus syndrome (CSS) is a condition which is defined by heart rate and blood pressure response to carotid sinus massage. The chances of developing carotid sinus hypersensitivity increase with age. Individuals with coronary artery disease or other heart conditions, hypertension, and head and neck tumors are more prone to develop this syndrome. Recent guidelines from European and American society of cardiology indicate that the criteria for CSS include a heart rate pause >3 seconds and a systolic blood pressure drop of >50 mm of Hg [49, 50]. Some have proposed to use the criteria of cerebral hypo perfusion for >5 seconds in the upright position [51]. Three types of CSS are seen: [1] cardio-inhibitory CSS, [2] vasodepressor CSS, and [3] mixed CSS. The diagnosis of CSS requires correct carotid sinus massage in the lying and upright position with continuous electrocardiogram (ECG) and blood pressure (BP) monitoring.

Vasovagal Syncope

Vasovagal syncope (VVS) is a condition where there is loss of consciousness due to decreased perfusion to the brain, with blood pressure drop and falling heart rate. In type 1 vasovagal syncope, with blood pressure falling before heart rate, and heart rate falling not below 40 beats per minute. Vasovagal syncope is the most common etiology of syncope. Head-up tilt test can be used to precipitate vasovagal syncope, as a diagnostic tool in patients with syncope of unknown etiology. A positive tilt table test suggests predisposition to VVS, but it does not provide a diagnosis of VVS by itself [52]. If the syncopal episode had normal sinus rhythm, it may be due to several disorders such as orthostatic hypotension, vasovagal or carotid sinus syndrome, or even psychogenic pseudo-syncope. With implantable loop recorders (ILR) one can do prolonged electrocardiographic monitoring and simultaneous suppression of both AV and sinus node activity which strongly suggests a diagnosis of VVS [53]. With a careful history focusing on predisposing situations, prodromal symptoms, physical signs, and recovery symptoms, the diagnosis of vasovagal syncope can be made correctly without further investigations. In elderly subjects up to 50% have atypical VVS without any triggers and a shorter or no prodrome and have amnesia for loss of consciousness but have a positive response to tilt testing [54, 55]. Tilt protocols are particularly useful for diagnosing atypical VVS and differentiating OH and syncope from seizures, as well as from psychogenic pseudo-syncope [56]. Reproducibility of VVS with tilt table testing protocols using sublingual nitroglycerine or intravenous isoproterenol is around 40–50% [57]. Recently a study by Kim et al. showed treadmill test with administration of sublingual nitroglycerines might be safely used to reproduce syncope in patients with VVS [58].

Post- exercise Hypotension

Post-exercise hypotension (PEH) is a condition where there is reduction in systolic and diastolic BP after exercise. Studies have used different criteria to define PEH. In some studies, PEH had been calculated as the difference between post- and pre-exercise BP (PEH I = post-exercise BP − pre-exercise BP) [59, 60]. In other studies, BP had been measured after an exercise and a control session, and PEH had been calculated as the difference between post-exercise and post-control BP (PEH II = post-exercise BP − post-control BP) [61], as well as the difference between the BP responses observed in the exercise and the control sessions [PEH III = (post-exercise BP − pre-exercise BP) − (post-control BP − pre-control BP)] [62]. In the study by Fecchio et al., systolic PEH had good/excellent reliability, while diastolic PEH had fair/poor reliability [63].

Nocturnal Hypotension

Dipping of the blood pressure in the night is a normal physiological change, and also extreme dipping or nocturnal hypotension is also seen in certain patients. Nocturnal hypotension can only be documented by 24-hour ambulatory blood pressure monitoring at this point. Nocturnal hypotension can be measured by nighttime dipping percentage (extreme dipper: an abnormal decrease in the nocturnal BP levels more than 20% in relation to diurnal BP levels) and by nighttime, daytime blood pressure ratio as suggested by Fagard et al. (Night/day BP ratios 0.8 indicate an extreme dipper) [64].

Challenges with Management

Symptom relief is the main focus in treating primary OH, not bringing it to a target BP value, such as the drop of SBP <20 or DBP <10 mm of Hg.

Non-pharmacological Management

Non-pharmacological interventions have been recommended as a first-line approach to treating OH. Goswami et al. suggested in addition to routine non-pharmacological measures to consider measures like mental challenge with arithmetic and cognitive training as well as respiratory training. Since the hemodynamic responses to mental challenge occur only for 2–3 minutes, it should be applied on symptomatic OH subjects upon standing up, to do mental arithmetic calculations starting before standing up and continuing for 2–3 minutes. This could increase sympathetic activity, improve venous return and cardiac output, and decrease blood pressure drop upon standing [65, 66]. Endothelium function affects vascular tone and may play a role in OH. Goswani et al. in their study showed cognitive training during bed rest does not improve endothelial function, but rather contributes to slowing down the impairment of endothelial function [67]. In a small, before-after intervention case-control study, Asian et al. showed inspiratory-expiratory pressure threshold respiratory training has reduced the incidence of orthostatic hypotension in more than 50% of patients with spinal cord injury [68]. Mechanisms related to increased sympathetic activation and baroreflex effectiveness are seen [69] (Table 9.2).

Pharmacological Management

OH: If conservative measures fail, pharmacotherapy can help ameliorate symptoms, including midodrine, droxidopa, fludrocortisone, pyridostigmine, atomoxetine, and sympathomimetic agents. Midodrine and droxidopa possess the most evidence with respect to increasing blood pressure and alleviating symptoms. Pharmacological therapy may be immediately added to the management in cases of symptomatic or severe OH. Emerging evidence with low-dose atomoxetine is promising, especially in those with central autonomic failure, and may prove to be a viable treatment option. When other medical treatment options have failed, atomoxetine may be a viable alternative. Atomoxetine raises BP dramatically even at small doses (18 mg) [70].

PPH: Eating smaller portions of low carbohydrate meals are tried to reduce symptomatic PPH. If patients are on anti-hypertensives, suggesting to change the timing of anti-hypertensive medications and avoiding their peak effects coincide with postprandial periods is recommended.

CSS: Treatment of vasodepressor CSS is not satisfactory and even for cardioinhibitory CSS, which can be treated with a pacemaker, syncope recurrence can occur in 5 years' time [71].

VSS: Medical interventions in the management of VVS have limited evidence with short-term trials, but long-term placebo-controlled trials are lacking [72–74].

Nocturnal hypotension: Applying the principles of chronotherapy of anti-hypertensive medications may help for a better preservation of normal physiological reductions at nighttime [75].

Table 9.2 Challenges with the Management of Hypotensive Syndromes

(a) Symptom relief is important, not bringing the BP to a target value.
(b) Cognitive and respiratory training for OH.
(c) Change anti-hypertensive timing in patients with high BP to avoid the peak effects coincide with postprandial periods.
(d) Long-term placebo-controlled medical trials are lacking for VVS.
(e) Chronotherapy of anti-hypertensive medications for preventing nocturnal hypotension.

Table 9.3 Drug
management of OH with
different co-morbid
conditions

OH + anemia = Erythropoietin
OH + renal failure = Erythropoietin, L-DOPS
Neurogenic OH = Midodrine, pyridostigmine, L-DOPS
OH + MSA = Octreotide, L-DOPS
OH + Parkinson's disease = L-DOPS or droxidopa
OH+ central autonomic failure = Atomoxetine

Adapted from Alagiakrishnan – Drugs and Aging 2015

Conclusions

Hypotensive syndromes are common conditions seen in the elderly. Many challenges with the measurement techniques of these hypotensive syndromes have to be addressed by future studies. Quality of outcome measures should be better studied in clinical trials related to hypotensive syndromes. One must also look beyond the numbers and evaluate the clinical presentation of each patient, because not all OHs are the same in terms of pathophysiology or approach to treatment. Current medication management of these symptomatic hypotensive syndromes remains suboptimal. Management should be individualized and concurrent illness should be considered (Table 9.3). Overtreatment of hypertension, especially in the frail elderly, can also result in these hypotensive syndromes like OH and PPH. Long-term follow-up medication studies are needed in older hypotensive adults.

References

1. The Consensus Committee of the American Autonomic Society and the American Academy of Neurology. Consensus statement on the definition of orthostatic hypotension, pure autonomic failure, and multiple system atrophy. Neurology. 1996;46:1470.
2. Streeten DH, Anderson GH Jr. Delayed orthostatic intolerance. Arch Intern Med. 1992;152:1066–72.
3. Ensrud KE, Nevitt MC, Yunis C, et al. Postural hypotension and postural dizziness in elderly women: the study of osteoporotic fractures. Arch Intern Med. 1992;152(5):1058–64.
4. Arbogast SD, Alshekhlee A, Huissain Z, et al. Hypotension unawareness in profound orthostatic hypotension. Am J Med. 2009;122(6):574–80.
5. Wieling W, Krediet CT, van Dijk N, et al. Initial orthostatic hypotension: review of a forgotten condition. Clin Sci (Lond). 2007;112:157–65.
6. Federowski A, Burri P, Melander O. Orthostatic hypotension in genetically related hypertensive and normotensive subjects. J Hypertension. 2009;27:976–82.
7. Wieling W, Schatz IJ. The consensus statement on the definition of orthostatic hypotension: a revisit after 13 years. J Hypertens. 2009;27(5):935–8.
8. Nwazue VC, Raj SR. Confounders of vasovagal syncope: Orthostatic hypotension. Cardiol Clin. 2013;31(1):89–100.
9. Alagiakrishnan K, Bu R, Hamilton P, et al. Comparison of the assessment of orthostatic hypotension using peripheral and central blood pressure measurements. J Clin Med Res. 2018;10(4):309–13.
10. Cheshire WP Jr. Clinical classification of orthostatic hypotension. Clin Auton Res. 2017;27:133–5.

11. Rutan GH, Hermanson B, Bild DE, Kittner SJ, LaBaw F, Tell GS. Orthostatic hypotension in older adults. The Cardiovascular Health Study. CHS Collaborative Research Group. Hypertension. 1992;19:508–19.
12. Fedorowski A, Melander O. Syndromes of orthostatic intolerance: a hidden danger. J Intern Med. 2013;273:322–35.
13. Freeman R, Wieling W, Axelrod FB, et al. Consensus statement on the definition of orthostatic hypotension, neurally mediated syncope and the postural tachycardia syndrome. Auton Neurosci. 2011;161(1–2):46–8.
14. Gibbons CH, Freeman R. Delayed orthostatic hypotension: a frequent cause of orthostatic intolerance. Neurology. 2006;67:28–32.
15. Grace Roy A, Gopinath S, Kumar S, et al. Delayed orthostatic hypotension: a pilot study from India. Ann Indian Acad Neurol. 2017;20(3):248–51.
16. Podoleanu C, Maggi R, Oddone D, et al. The hemodynamic pattern of the syndrome of delayed orthostatic hypotension. J Interv Card Electrophysiol. 2009;26(2):143–9.
17. Madhavan G, Goddard AA, McLeod KJ. Prevalence and etiology of delayed orthostatic hypotension in adult women. Arch Phys Med Rehabil. 2008;89(9):1788–94.
18. Freeman R. Clinical practice. Neurogenic orthostatic hypotension. N Engl J Med. 2008;358:615–24.
19. Gibbons CH, Freeman R. Orthostatic dyspnea: a neglected symptom of orthostatic hypotension. Clin Auton Res. 2005;15:40–4.
20. Gibbons CH, Freeman R. Clinical implications of delayed orthostatic hypotension. A 10-year follow-up study. Neurology. 2015;85(16):1362–7.
21. Lee J, Salathé EP, Schmid-Schönbein GW. Fluid exchange in skeletal muscle with viscoelastic blood vessels. Am J Phys. 1987;253(6. Pt 2):H1548–56.
22. Vito RP, Dixon SA. Blood vessel constitutive models—1995–2002. Annu Rev Biomed Eng. 2003;5:413–39.
23. Hagan RD, Diaz FJ, Horvath SM. Plasma volume changes with movement to supine and standing positions. J Appl Physiol. 1978;45:414–7.
24. Joyner MJ, Shepherd JT, Seals DR. Sustained increases in sympathetic outflow during prolonged lower body negative pressure in humans. J Appl Physiol. 1990;68:1004–9.
25. Gloviczki P, Yao J. Handbook of venous disorders: guidelines of the American venous forum. 2nd ed. London: Hodder Arnold Publication; 2001.
26. Stewart JM, Karman C, Montgomery LD, McLeod KJ. Plantar vibration improves leg fluid flow in perimenopausal women. Am J Physiol Regul Integr Comp Physiol. 2005;288:R623–9.
27. Fedorowski A, Van Wijnen VK, Wieling W. Delayed orthostatic hypotension and vasovagal syncope: a diagnostic dilemma. Clin Auton Res. 2017;27:289–91.
28. Gurevich T, Machmid H, Klepikov D, et al. Head-up tilt testing for detecting orthostatic hypotension: how long do we need to wait? Neuroepidemiology. 2014;43(3–4):239–43.
29. Belmin J, Abderrhamane M, Medjahed S, et al. Variability of blood pressure response to orthostatism and reproducibility of the diagnosis of orthostatic hypotension in elderly subjects. J Gerontol A Biol Sci Med Sci. 2000;55(11):M667–71.
30. Ward C, Kenny RA. Reproducibility of orthostatic hypotension in symptomatic elderly. Am J Med. 1996;100(4):418–22.
31. Weiss A, Grossman E, Beloosesky Y, et al. Orthostatic hypotension in acute geriatric ward: is it a consistent finding? Arch Intern Med. 2002;162:2369–74.
32. O'Brien E. A century of confusion: which bladder for accurate blood pressure measurement? J Hum Hypertension. 1996;10:565–72.
33. O'Brien E, Petrie J, Littler WA, et al. Blood pressure measurement: recommendations of the British Hypertension Society. 3rd ed. London: BMJ Publishing Group; 1997.
34. Benrud-Larson LM, Dewar MS, Sandroni P, et al. Quality of life in patients with postural tachycardia syndrome. Mayo Clin Proc. 2002;77(6):531–7.
35. Naschitz JE, Rosner I. Orthostatic hypotension: framework of the syndrome. Postgrad Med J. 2007;83:568–74.

36. Cooke J, Carew S, O'Connor M, et al. Sitting and standing blood pressure measurements are not accurate for the diagnosis of orthostatic hypotension. QJM. 2009;102(5):335–9.
37. Tabara Y, Nakura J, Kondo I, et al. Orthostatic systolic hypotension and the reflection pressure wave. Hypertens Res. 2005;28(6):537–43.
38. Jansen RW, Lipsitz LA. Postprandial hypotension: epidemiology, pathophysiology, and clinical management. Ann Intern Med. 1995;122(4):286–95.
39. Narender P, Van Orshoven J, Paul AF, et al. Postprandial hypotension in clinical geriatric patients and healthy elderly: prevalence related to patient selection and diagnostic criteria. J Aging Res. 2010;2010:243752.
40. Aronow WS, Ahn C. Postprandial hypotension in 499 elderly persons in a long-term health care facility. J Am Geriatr Soc. 1994;42(9):930–2.
41. Jansen RWMM, Kelley-Gagnon MM, Lipsitz LA. Intraindividual reproducibility of postprandial and orthostatic blood pressure changes in older nursing-home patients: relationship with chronic use of cardiovascular medications. J Am Geriatr Soc. 1996;44(4):383–9.
42. Kohara K, Uemura K, Takata Y, et al. Postprandial hypotension: evaluation by ambulatory blood pressure monitoring. Am J Hypertens. 1998;11(11 I):1358–63.
43. Puisieux F, Bulckaen H, Fauchais AL, et al. Ambulatory blood pressure monitoring and postprandial hypotension in elderly persons with falls or syncopes. J Gerontol A. 2000;55(9):M535–40.
44. Imai C, Muratani H, Kimura Y, et al. Effects of meal ingestion and active standing on blood pressure in patients ≤60 years of age. Am J Cardiol. 1998;81(11):1310–4.
45. Maurer MS, Karmally W, Rivadeneira H, et al. Upright posture and postprandial hypotension in elderly persons. Ann Intern Med. 2000;133(7):533–6.
46. Pulsieux F, Court D, Baheu E, et al. Intraindividual reproducibility of postprandial hypotension. Gerontology. 2002;48(5):315–20.
47. Alfie J. Utility of home blood pressure monitoring to evaluate postprandial blood pressure in treated hypertensive patients. Ther Adv Cardiovasc Dis. 2015;9(4):133–9.
48. Abbas R, Tanguy A, Bonnet-Zamponi D, et al. New simplified screening method for postprandial hypotension in older people. J Frailty Aging. 2018;7(1):28–33.
49. Shen WK, Sheldon RS, Benditt DG, et al. 2017 ACC/AHA/HRS guideline for the evaluation and management of patients with syncope: a report of the American College of Cardiology/American Heart Association Task Force on Clinical Practice Guidelines, and the Heart Rhythm Society. J Am Coll Cardiol. 2017;70(5):620–63.
50. Brignole M, Moya A, de Lange FJ, et al. ESC guidelines for the diagnosis and management of syncope. Eur Heart J 2018. 2018;39:1883.
51. Krediet CT, Parry SW, Jardine DL, et al. The history of diagnosing carotid sinus hypersensitivity: why are the current criteria too sensitive? Europace. 2011;13:14.
52. Chew DS, Raj SR, Sheldon RS. Vasovagal syncope in 2016: the current state of the faint. Arrhythm Open Access. 2016;1:117. https://doi.org/10.4172/atoa.1000117.
53. Brignole M, Menozzi C, Moya A, Andresen D, Blanc JJ, et al. Pacemaker therapy in patients with neurally mediated syncope and documented asystole: Third International Study on Syncope of Uncertain Etiology (ISSUE-3): a randomized trial. Circulation. 2012;125:2566–71.
54. Alboni P. The different clinical presentations of vasovagal syncope. Heart. 2015;10:674–8.
55. O'Dwyer C, Bennett K, Langan Y, et al. Amnesia for loss of consciousness is common in vasovagal syncope. Europace. 2011;13:1040–5.
56. Forleo C, Guida P, Iacoviello M, et al. Head-up tilt testing for diagnosing vasovagal syncope: a meta-analysis. Int J Cardiol. 2013;169:e49–50.
57. Raviele A, Giada F, Brignole M, et al. Comparison of diagnostic accuracy of sublingual nitroglycerin test and low-dose isoproterenol test in patients with unexplained syncope. Am J Cardiol. 2000;85:1194–8.
58. Kim T-H, Jang H-J, Kim S, et al. A new test for diagnosing vasovagal syncope: standing after treadmill test with sublingual nitrate administration. PLoS One. 2017;12(6):e0179631.
59. Santaella DF, Araújo EA, Ortega KC, et al. After effects of exercise and relaxation on blood pressure. Clin J Sport Med. 2006;16:341–7.

60. Forjaz CL, Santaella DF, Rezende LO, et al. Effect of exercise duration on the magnitude and duration of post-exercise hypotension. Arq Bras Cardiol. 1998;70:99–104.
61. Jones H, George K, Edwards B, et al. Is the magnitude of acute post-exercise hypotension mediated by exercise intensity or total work done? Eur J Appl Physiol. 2007;102:33–40.
62. Lacombe SP, Goodman JM, Spragg CM, et al. Interval and continuous exercise elicit equivalent post-exercise hypotension in prehypertensive men, despite differences in regulation. Appl Physiol Nutr Metab. 2011;36:881–91.
63. Fecchio RY, Chehuen M, Brito LC, et al. Reproducibility/reliability and agreement of post-exercise hypotension. Int J Sports Med. 2017;38(13):1029–34.
64. Fagard R, Thijs L, Staessen JA, et al. Night and day blood pressure ratio and dipping pattern as predictors of death and cardiovascular events in hypertension. J Hum Hypertens. 2009;23:645–53.
65. Goswami N, Lackner HK, Papousek I, et al. Does mental arithmetic before head up tilt have an effect on the orthostatic cardiovascular and hormonal responses? Acta Astronaut. 2011;68:1589–94.
66. Goswami N, Blaber AP, Hinghofer-Szalkay H, et al. Orthostatic intolerance in older persons: etiology and countermeasures. Front Physiol. 2017;8:803. https://doi.org/10.3389/fphys.2017.00803.
67. Goswani N, Kavcic V, Marusic V, et al. Effect of computerised cognitive training with virtual spatial navigation task during bed rest immobilization and recovery on vascular function: a pilot study. Clin Interv Aging. 2015;10:453–9.
68. Asian SC, Randall DC, Krassioukov AV, et al. Respiratory training improves blood pressure regulation in individuals with chronic spinal cord injury. Arch Phys Med Rehabil. 2016;97(6):964–73.
69. Legg Ditterline BE, Asian SC, Randall DC, et al. Effects of respiratory training and heart rate variability and baroreflex sensitivity in individuals with chronic spinal cord injury. Arch Phys Med Rehabil. 2018;99(3):423–32.
70. Hale GM, Valdes J, Brenner M. The treatment of primary orthostatic hypotension. Ann Pharmacother. 2017;51(5):417–28.
71. Sutton R. Carotid sinus syndrome: progress in understanding and management. Glob Cardiol Sci Pract. 2014;2014(2):1–8.
72. Sheldon RS, Morillo CA, Klingenheben T, et al. Age-dependent effect of beta-blockers in preventing vasovagal syncope. Circ Arrhythm Electrophysiol. 2012;5:920–6.
73. Sheldon R, Raj SR, Rose MS. Fludrocortisone for the prevention of vasovagal syncope: a randomized, placebo-controlled trial. J Am Coll Cardiol. 2016;68:1–9.
74. Izcovich A, González Malla C, Manzotti M, et al. Midodrine for orthostatic hypotension and recurrent reflex syncope: a systematic review. Neurology. 2014;83:1170–7.
75. Hermida RC, Ayala DE, Fontao MJ, et al. Chronotherapy with valsartan/amlodipine fixed combination: improved blood pressure control of essential hypertension with bedtime dosing. Chronobiol Int. 2010;27(6):1287–303.

Hypertension and Hypotensive Syndromes

10

Kannayiram Alagiakrishnan

Introduction

Autonomic control of blood pressure is essential towards maintenance of cerebral perfusion and perfusion to other organs. Autonomic dysfunction in elderly hypertensives may contribute to different hypotensive syndromes associated with hypertension.

Hypertension and Orthostatic Hypotension

Hypertension and orthostatic hypotension (OH) is seen together in elderly subjects. With aging, the incidence of both conditions increases. It was seen in 10% of subjects referred to the hypertension clinic [1]. With aging, baroreflex and autonomic function changes occur which can contribute to OH. Uncontrolled hypertension, use of three or more antihypertensive medications and multiple co-morbidities are predictors of OH in older women [2]. Elderly with uncontrolled hypertension have more incidence of OH and in this group there was also two-fold increase in falls [3].

Healthcare providers always face the management challenge of hypotension in hypertensive subjects. Observational studies had found the use of diuretics, alpha blockers, central sympatholytics and beta blockers are associated with OH, but no association was seen with calcium channel blockers, angiotensin-converting enzyme (ACE) inhibitors and angiotensin receptor blockers (ARB) [1, 2, 4]. In patients with hypertension, better control of hypertension reduced hypotensive episodes [5]. Coexistence of hypertension with OH complicates the management of both conditions, as the treatment of one can worsen the other.

10

K. Alagiakrishnan (✉)
Division of Geriatric Medicine, University of Alberta, Edmonton, AB, Canada

© Springer Nature Switzerland AG 2020
K. Alagıakrıshnan, M. Banach (eds.), *Hypotensive Syndromes in Geriatric Patients*, https://doi.org/10.1007/978-3-030-30332-7_10

Clinical Outcomes of OH in Hypertensive Subjects

OH in hypertension, may be symptomatic or asymptomatic like seen in normotensives. Common symptoms include dizziness, light-headedness, blurred vision, syncope and falls. In Boston study of the elderly, uncontrolled hypertension and OH can increase the risk of falls two-fold [3]. Natriuresis, nocturia and autonomic dysfunction contribute to hypertension and OH in these conditions [6].

Management of OH with Hypertension

Symptom relief is the main focus when treating primary OH. Non-pharmacological interventions have been recommended as a first-line approach to treat OH. Pharmacological therapy may be immediately added to these interventions in cases of severe or symptomatic OH [7]. When other medical treatment options for OH have failed, atomoxetine may be a viable alternative. Atomoxetine raises BP dramatically at small doses, specifically at 18 mg. Atomoxetine significantly raises seated and standing BP [8].

In the Epicardian study of 2700 elderly subjects, the incidence of OH with adequate control of blood pressure was low [5]. Another prospective study of older adults with hypertension had demonstrated an improvement in postural blood pressure changes with antihypertensive medications [9]. Vasodilators (alpha-adrenoceptor antagonists), diuretics and certain short-acting calcium channel blockers can exacerbate postural blood pressure changes, whereas beta-blockers with intrinsic sympathomimetic activity, ACE inhibitors, long-acting calcium channel blockers and angiotensin receptor antagonists are less likely to worsen postural changes [10]. For individuals who experience OH with hypertension, management should aim for adequate treatment of hypertension and avoidance of antihypertensive medications that cause OH (Table 10.1).

If multiple antihypertensive medications are causing OH, consider stopping or tapering one medication at a time. Check for medications used for other conditions that can also contribute to OH. Labetalol which has combined alpha and beta blocking properties can also give rise to OH [11]. Slavachevsky et al. in their cross-over study found that enalapril reduces the episodes of OH when compared to long-acting nifedipine, even though they had equal potency in reducing supine blood pressure levels [12].

Hypertension and Postprandial Hypotension (PPH)

Studies have shown that the occurrence of PPH is seen among individuals with essential and isolated systolic hypertension [13, 14]. Whereas in essential hypertensive patients, PPH was also associated with asymptomatic cerebrovascular damage [15]. A recent study by Zhang et al. showed the prevalence of PPH was 19% in subjects with essential hypertension and coronary heart disease, and the baseline

Table 10.1 Medications causing OH and possible alternatives

Medications	Alternatives
1. Antihypertensives	
Alpha blockers:	
Doxazosin	Long-acting CCB, ACEI, ARB
Combined alpha and beta blockers:	
Labetalol	
Diuretics:	
Furosemide, hydrochlorothiazide	
2. BPH medications:	
Tamsulosin	Finasteride
3. Antidepressants:	
TCA	SSRI, SNRI

CCB calcium channel blockers, *ACEI* angiotensin-converting enzyme inhibitors, *ARB* angiotensin receptor blockers, *TCA* tricyclic antidepressants, *SSRI* selective serotonin reuptake inhibitors, *SNRI* serotonin and norepinephrine reuptake inhibitors

systolic blood pressure was considered to be the risk factor of PPH in this study. Authors suggested that PPH could lead to an increase of major adverse cardiac and cerebral vascular events in these subjects [16]. A study on 578 European subjects who were included in the SYST-EUR trial had their ambulatory blood pressure monitoring (ABPM) done, and in 25% of subjects who had isolated systolic hypertension and postprandial fall in blood pressure, a decrease of more than 16 mm of Hg in SBP or 12 mmHg in DBP had occurred [14]. Home blood pressure monitoring (HBPM) using premeal and post-meal measurements may be used to evaluate the effect of food on blood pressure. Home blood pressure self-monitoring could be a suitable screening test for PPH in hypertensive subjects [17, 18]. HBPM offers a number of advantages over ABPM: easier to perform, can be evaluated after different meals over different days, cheaper and may be guiding treatment adjustments according to the blood pressure response. In another study, isolated morning hypertension in treated hypertensive subjects who underwent home blood measurements was associated with meal-induced blood pressure fall [19].

Clinical Outcomes of PPH in Hypertension

Postprandial hypotension may be a source of visit-to-visit blood pressure variability and masked hypertension when the clinical appointment takes place during the subsequent hours after a meal [20]. Even smaller declines in systolic blood pressure (SBP) after meals (10–20 mmHg) as detected by ambulatory blood pressure monitoring (ABPM), were associated with greater number of lacunar infarction in middle-aged to elderly persons from the community [21]. In the study by Barochiner et al., higher systolic BP by office blood pressure monitoring was a risk factor for PPH in hypertensive subjects [17]. In a prospective cohort study on ambulatory patients, using 24-hour ABPM, a diurnal standard deviation of SBP of 10 mmHg or higher was predictive of PPH, with a sensitivity and specificity of 87% and 57%, respectively. This study also showed breakfast blood pressure as a possible new risk factor for cardiovascular mortality [22]. Masuo et al. showed in their study that in hypertensive patients, subjects with orthostatic hypotension were only prone to develop postprandial hypotension and the pathophysiology of postprandial and orthostatic hypotension were similar [23].

In a small case-control study by Shimosawa et al. PPH was commonly seen in hypertensive subjects compared to normotensive subjects, and impairment of the sympathetic nervous system in the elderly with hypertension was involved in the mechanism of PPH [24, 25].

Management of PPH with Hypertension

Patients with postprandial hypotension should be advised to avoid high-carbohydrate meals [26]. In the study by Alfie et al., the prevalence of postprandial hypotension was 13.2% in controlled and 42.2% in uncontrolled hypertensive patients (p < 0.001) and the need for adjustments in antihypertensive treatment according to postprandial blood pressure [18]. In another cohort study by Mitro et al., PPH was detected in 45% of subjects with arterial hypertension and greater postprandial reduction in blood pressure was seen in subjects who were using diuretics [13]. Adequate treatment of hypertension and avoidance of diuretics can help to reduce the postprandial blood pressure drop.

Hypertension and Post-Exercise Hypotension

Studies have shown the effect of exercise on blood pressure lowering effect as well as post-exercise hypotension (PEH) [27, 28]. In a study by Domingos et al., resistance exercise with blood flow restriction resulted in greater post-exercise hypotension than traditional exercise in hypertensive individuals [29].

Hypertension with Vasovagal Syndrome

Limited information in the literature about these two conditions occurring together. It could be neurocardiovascular disorders (NCVD) with sympathetically mediated condition, where both hypertension and hypotension can occur together. VVS types cause an enhancement of the vagal system and withdrawal of sympathetic system, but mixed types can also occur [30].

Hypertension with Carotid Sinus Syndrome

No information was available in the literature about these conditions together. Future research is needed.

Hypertension and Nocturnal Hypotension

Dipping of the blood pressure in the night is a normal physiological change seen in both normotensives and hypertensives. Healthcare professionals concentrate on daytime blood pressure, but not on nighttime blood pressure values [31]. The dipping pattern and the night-day BP ratio significantly and independently predicted mortality and cardiovascular events in hypertensive patients [32]. Extreme dippers or nocturnal hypotension is prevalent in 4–20% of subjects with hypertension. In this meta-analysis study, extreme dippers had an increased risk of total Cardiovascular (CV) events compared to normally dipping hypertensive patients [33]. Kario et al. in their study showed increased risk of cerebrovascular damage [34]. Nocturnal hypotension is a risk factor for hypertensive target organ damage and cardiovascular events as well as risk of cerebrovascular disease. Extreme-dippers or nocturnal hypotension is at risk for non-fatal ischemic stroke and silent myocardial ischemia, particularly with excessive BP reduction when on antihypertensive medications. Nocturnal hypotension was closely associated with excessive morning BP surge and orthostatic hypertension [35]. Recent evidence suggests that some patients may be adversely affected by excessive lowering of nocturnal BP that causes decreased perfusion to the brain and the heart [36, 37]. Chronotherapy with antihypertensive medications reduces the side effect and optimizes the benefits of blood pressure lowering medications at nighttime [38, 39].

The effect of chronotherapy in achieving overall BP control for combination of valsartan and amlodipine was also studied. "For instance, 203 hypertensives were randomized to a combination of valsartan and amlodipine either in the morning or night, in one of the four combinations. Forty-eight hour mean systolic and diastolic BP were reduced significantly when both were given in the night compared to other combinations. The reduction was 17.4/13.4 mmHg with both medications on awakening; 15.1/9.6 mmHg with valsartan on awakening and amlodipine at bedtime; 18.2/12.3 mmHg with valsartan at bedtime and amlodipine on awakening; and 24.7/13.5 mmHg with both medications administered at bedtime (P < 0.018 between groups). This study established that for a given dose and combination of antihypertensives, administering them in the night results in better reduction of nocturnal BP than when they are given in the morning" [40].

Chronotherapy of Hypertension

Chronobiology is the science related to biological rhythms. Chronotherapy helps to individualize antihypertensive treatment according to circadian blood pressure changes. The chronotherapy of hypertension is a relatively new practice. When nighttime blood pressure goal of <120/ 70 mm of Hg is achieved, there is more likely possibility of preventing major cardiovascular and cerebrovascular events (Orías M, Correa-Rotter R. Chronotherapy in hypertension: a pill at night makes things right? *J Am Soc Nephrol* 2011; 22 [11]:2152–2155). In order to achieve this, there is a need to use the 24-hour ambulatory BP monitoring not just only for diagnosis, but also for monitoring. The chronotherapy of hypertension not only reduces the risks associated with hypertension but also has the potential of reducing the effects of hypotensive syndromes.

Conclusions

Different hypotensive syndromes are seen in patients with hypertension. Ambulatory blood pressure monitoring can help to diagnose these hypotensive syndromes. Screening for symptomatic and asymptomatic hypotensive syndromes should be done in hypertensive subjects. In subjects with hypertension and hypotensive syndromes, non-pharmacological methods should be considered in addition to control hypertension with preferable antihypertensives, which can also reduce hypotensive syndrome episodes in the elderly.

In patients with hypertension and OH, healthcare providers should not hold antihypertensive treatment, but control hypertension with preferable antihypertensives like ARB, ACEI and CCB, but avoid alpha blockers, diuretics and central sympatholytics. Adequate treatment of hypertension and avoidance of diuretics can help to reduce the postprandial blood pressure drop in hypertensive subjects. Future research may help us to better understand these conditions as well as the therapeutic modalities.

References

1. Di Stefano C, Milazzo V, Totaro S, et al. Orthostatic hypotension in a cohort of hypertensive patients referring to a hypertension clinic. J Hum Hypertens. 2015;29:599–603.
2. Kamaruzzaman S, Watt H, Carson C, et al. The association between orthostatic hypotension and medication use in the British Women's Heart and Health Study. Age Ageing. 2010;39:51–6.
3. Gangavati A, Hajjar I, Quach L, et al. Hypertension, orthostatic hypotension, and the risk of falls in a community-dwelling elderly population: the maintenance of balance, independent living, intellect, and zest in the elderly of Boston study. J Am Geriatr Soc. 2011;59:383–9.
4. Canney M, O'Connell MD, Murphy CM, et al. Single agent antihypertensive therapy and orthostatic blood pressure behaviour in older adults using beat-to-beat measurements: the Irish Longitudinal Study on Ageing. PLoS One. 2016;11:e0146156.
5. Saez T, Suarez C, Sierra MJ, et al. Orthostatic hypotension in the aged and its association with antihypertensive treatment. Med Clin (Barc). 2000;114:525–9.
6. Jordan J, Shannon JR, Pohar B, et al. Contrasting effects of vasodilators on blood pressure and sodium balance in the hypertension of autonomic failure. J Am Soc Nephrol. 1999;10:35–42.
7. Jones PK, Shaw BH, Raj SR. Orthostatic hypotension: managing a difficult problem. Expert Rev Cardiovasc Ther. 2015;13:1263–76.
8. Patel H, Simpson A, Palevoda G, Hale GM. Evaluating the effectiveness of atomoxetine for the treatment of primary orthostatic hypotension in adults. J Clin Hypertens. 2018;20:794–7.
9. Masuo K, Mikami H, Ogihara T, et al. Changes in frequency of orthostatic hypotension in elderly hypertensive patients under medications. Am J Hypertens. 1996;9:263–8.
10. Hajjar I. Postural blood pressure changes and orthostatic hypotension in the elderly patient: impact of antihypertensive medications. Drugs Aging. 2006;22:55–68.
11. Pearce CJ, Wallin JD. Labetalol and other agents that block both alpha and beta-adrenergic receptors. Cleve Clin J Med. 1994;61(1):59–69.

12. Slavachevsky I, Rachmani R, Levi Z, et al. Effect of enalapril and nifedipine on orthostatic hypotension in older hypertensive patients. J Am Geriatr Soc. 2000;48(7):807–10.
13. Mitro P, Feterik K, Cverckova A, et al. Occurrence and relevance of postprandial hypotension in patients with essential hypertension. Wien Klin Wochenschr. 1999;111:320–5.
14. Grodzicki T, Rajzer M, Fagard R, et al. Ambulatory blood pressure monitoring and postprandial hypotension in elderly patients with isolated systolic hypertension. J Hum Hypertens. 1998;12:161–5.
15. Kohara K, Jiang Y. Postprandial hypotension is associated with asymptomatic cerebrovascular damage in essential hypertensive patients. Hypertension. 1999;33:565–8.
16. Zhang YN, Tl C, Geng X, et al. Clinical observation of postprandial hypotension in patients with hypertensive and coronary artery disease. Zhonghua Yi Xue Za Zhi. 2018;98(33):2641–4.
17. Barochiner J, Alfie J, Aparicio L, et al. Postprandial hypotension detected through home blood pressure monitoring: a frequent phenomenon in elderly hypertensive patients. Hypertens Res. 2014;37:438–43.
18. Alfie J. Utility of home blood pressure monitoring to evaluate postprandial blood pressure in treated hypertensive subjects. Ther Adv Cardiovasc Dis. 2015;9(4):133–9.
19. Barochiner J, Alfie J, Aparicio LS, et al. Meal induced blood pressure fall in patients with isolated morning hypertension. Clin Exp Hypertens. 2015;37(5):364–8.
20. Fagan T, Conrad K, Mar J, et al. Effects of meals on hemodynamics: implications for antihypertensive drug studies. Clin Pharmacol Ther. 1986;39:255–60.
21. Tabara Y, Okada Y, Uetani E, et al. Postprandial hypotension as a risk marker for asymptomatic lacunar infarction. J Hypertens. 2014;32:1084–90.
22. Zanasi A, Tincani E, Evandri V, et al. Meal induced blood pressure variation and cardiovascular mortality in ambulatory hypertensive elderly patients: preliminary results. J Hypertens. 2012;30:2125–32.
23. Masuo K, Mikami H, Habara N, et al. Orthostatic and postprandial blood pressure reduction in patients with essential hypertension. Clin Exp Pharmacol Physiol. 1991;18:155–61.
24. Shimosawa T, Kuwajima I, Suzuki Y, et al. Postprandial hypotension in the elderly with and without hypertension. Nihon Ronen Igakkai Zasshi. 1992;29(9):661–6.
25. Haigh RA, Harper GD, Burton R, et al. Possible impairment of the sympathetic nervous system response to postprandial hypotension in elderly hypertensive patients. J Hum Hypertens. 1991;5:83–9.
26. Teunissen-Beekman K, Dopheide J, Geleijnse J, et al. Blood pressure decreases more after high-carbohydrate meals than after high-protein meals in overweight adults with elevated blood pressure, but there is no difference after 4 weeks of consuming a carbohydrate-rich or protein-rich diet. J Nutr. 2013;143:424–9.
27. Casonatto J, Goessler KF, Cornelissen VA, et al. The blood pressure-lowering effect of a single bout of resistance exercise: a systematic review and meta-analysis of randomised controlled trials. Eur J Prev Cardiol. 2016;23:1700–14.
28. MacDonald HV, Johnson BT, Huedo-Medina TB, et al. Dynamic resistance training as stand-alone antihypertensive lifestyle therapy: a meta-analysis. J Am Heart Assoc. 2016;5(10) https://doi.org/10.1161/JAHA.116.003231. pii: e003231.
29. Domingos E, Politio MD. Blood pressure response between resistance exercise with and without blood flow restriction: A systematic review and meta-analysis. Life Sci. 2018;209:122–31.
30. Fisher JP, Paton JF. The sympathetic nervous system and blood pressure in humans: implications for hypertension. J Hum Hypertens. 2011;26:463–75.
31. Friedman O, Logan AG. Nocturnal blood pressure profiles among normotensive, controlled hypertensive and refractory hypertensive subjects. Can J Cardiol. 2009;25(9):S312–6.
32. Fagard R, Thijs L, Staessen JA, et al. Night and day blood pressure ratio and dipping pattern as predictors of death and cardiovascular events in hypertension. J Hum Hypertens. 2009;23:645–53.
33. Salles GF, Reboldi G, Fagard RH, et al. Prognostic effect of the nocturnal blood pressure fall in hypertensive patients: the ambulatory blood pressure collaboration in patients with hypertension (ABC-H) meta-analysis. Hypertension. 2016;67(4):693–700.

34. Kario K, Shimada K. Risers and extreme-dippers of nocturnal blood pressure in hypertension: antihypertensive strategy for nocturnal blood pressure. Clin Exp Hypertens. 2004;26(2):177–89.
35. Fagard RH. Dipping pattern of nocturnal blood pressure in patients with hypertension. Expert Rev Cardiovasc Ther. 2009;7:599–605.
36. Benetos A, Bulpitt CJ, Petrovic M, et al. An expert opinion from the European society of hypertension-European union geriatric medicine society working group on the management of hypertension in very old, frail subjects. Hypertension. 2016;67:820–5.
37. O'Brien E, Kario K, Staessen JA, et al. Patterns of ambulatory blood pressure: clinical relevance and application. J Clin Hypertension. 2018;20(7):1112–5.
38. Fujiwara T, Hoshide S, Yano Y, et al. Comparison of morning vs bedtime administration of the combination of valsartan/amlodipine on nocturnal brachial and central blood pressure in patients with hypertension. J Clin Hypertens (Greenwich). 2017;19:1319–26.
39. Bowles NP, Thosar SS, Herzig MX, et al. Chronotherapy for hypertension. Curr Hypertens Rep. 2018;20:11.
40. Hermida RC, Ayala DE, Fontao MJ, et al. Chronotherapy with valsartan/amlodipine fixed combination: improved blood pressure control of essential hypertension with bedtime dosing. Chronobiol Int. 2010;27(6):1287–303.

Diabetes Mellitus

11

Paulina Gorzelak-Pabiś and Marlena Broncel

Introduction

In a patient with diabetes, cardiovascular autonomic neuropathy (CAN) is a risk marker and probably a risk factor for cardiovascular morbidity, as well as a risk marker of mortality. The reported prevalence of CAN in clinic-based studies including both type 1 and type 2 diabetic patients varied from 16.6 to 20%. However, prevalence rates increased with age, up to 38% in type 1 and 44% in type 2 patients aged 40–70 years, and with diabetes duration, up to 35% in type 1 and 65% in type 2 patients with long-standing diabetes [6]. Together with postural hypotension, postprandial hypotension, orthostatic tachycardia and bradycardia syndromes, exercise intolerance, and silent myocardial ischemia (cardiac denervation syndrome), orthostatic hypotension (OH) is one of the major clinical signs of cardiovascular autonomic neuropathy (CAN) [3, 4]. The results of 15 different studies found the pooled estimated relative mortality risk to be 3.45 (95% CI 2.66–4.47, P < 0.001) where CAN was defined as the presence of two or more abnormalities in cardiac autonomic function in patients with diabetes [9]. The Action to Control Cardiovascular Risk in Diabetes (ACCORD) trial showed CAN to be an independent predictor of all-cause mortality (HR 2.14, 95% CI 1.37–3.37) and Cardiovascular disease (CVD) mortality (HR 2.62, 95% CI 1.4–4.91) after a mean follow-up of 3.5 years [10]. Symptomatic CAN at 5 years of diabetes predicted mortality at 10 years, even after adjusting for conventional CVD risk factors. In addition, clinic-based studies of 1319 patients with type 1 diabetes and 3396 patients with type 2 diabetes, with a mean follow-up of 9.2 years, found QT interval (QTi) prolongation to be an independent predictor of mortality for all-cause and cardiovascular deaths [10, 11].

P. Gorzelak-Pabiś (✉) · M. Broncel
Department of Internal Diseases and Clinical Pharmacology, Medical University of Lodz, Lodz, Poland

© Springer Nature Switzerland AG 2020
K. Alagiakrishnan, M. Banach (eds.), *Hypotensive Syndromes in Geriatric Patients*, https://doi.org/10.1007/978-3-030-30332-7_11

Pathomechanism

The pathogenesis of CAN is complex and remains unclear. CAN is believed to occur as a result of abnormalities in heart rate control caused by damage to the autonomic nerve fibers that innervate the heart and blood vessels; the mechanism is thought to be due to neuronal injury caused by somatic neuropathy. Although somatic neuropathy and autonomic neuropathy are similar in many respects, the Steno-2 trial found that multifactorial intervention can prevent the progression of autonomic neuropathy but not somatic neuropathy [13].

Hyperglycemia, autoimmune autonomic ganglionopathy, inflammation, and obstructive sleep apnea can all activate multiple pathways involved in the pathogenesis of CAN.

Hyperglycemia can cause mitochondrial dysfunction and the formation of reactive oxygen species (ROS). Increased ROS is thought to influence CAN by depressing autonomic ganglion synaptic transmission, thus contributing to an increased risk of fatal cardiac arrhythmias, as well as to sudden death after myocardial infarction, due to posttranslational protein modifications. Glycemic control is considered an essential component of treating CAN [14].

Autoimmune autonomic ganglionopathy is where autonomic failure occurs in the presence of antibodies to the nicotinic acetylcholine receptor of the autonomic ganglia, leading to a range of severe autonomic manifestations, including orthostatic intolerance, syncope, constipation, and gastroparesis [15]. However, the role of autoimmunity in patients with diabetes and CAN remains unclear.

CAN has also been associated with increased levels of *inflammatory markers* such as CRP, IL-6, TNFa, and adipose tissue inflammation. The pathogenesis of micro- and macrovascular complications has been associated with inflammatory processes, but the relationship between inflammation and CAN remains unclear [16].

Obstructive sleep apnea(OSA) has also been found to be linked to CAN; this relationship is believed to be associated with intermittent hypoxia that results in increased ROS and impaired microvascular function. The pathophysiology of obstructive sleep apnea and CAN may differ between patients with type 1 DM and type 2 DM [17]. Janovsky et al. showed that while OSA was common in non-obese patients with type 1 DM, it was most likely associated with Diabetic peripheral neuropathy (DPN) in patients with type 2 DM [6].

Diagnosis

Cardiac autonomic reflex tests (CARTs) are gold-standard measures of autonomic function, as they are non-invasive, safe, relatively easy to perform, sensitive, specific, reproducible, and standardized. Tests such as heart rate variations (HRV) during deep breathing (E:I ratio - expiration/inspiration), Valsalva maneuver (Valsalva ratio), and lying-to-standing (HR response to standing - 30:15 ratio) are mainly indices of parasympathetic function, whereas the OH test (BP response to standing - reduction in SBP), the blood pressure response to a Valsalva maneuver, and sustained isometric muscular strain (BP response to sustained muscle contraction - rise in DBP) provide indices of sympathetic function [23]. The *defined CAN* is defined as the presence of at least two abnormal CARTs, possible or *early CAN* is regarded as the presence of one abnormal CART, while *severe* or *advanced CAN* is indicated by the presence of orthostatic hypotension with two or more abnormal CARTs.

Progressive stages of CAN are associated with increasingly worse prognosis [3] (Fig. 11.1).

Treatment

CAN is treated by symptom control or slowing its progression. Current methods use a combination of nonpharmacological and pharmacological approaches.

It should also be remembered that despite their similarities, CAN and DPN are not the same disease, and they demonstrate different responses to treatment. Diabetic patients with CAN can receive nonpharmacological interventions including lifestyle modification, intensive glycemic control, and treatment of risk factors such as hyperlipidemia and hypertension [13]. A number of drugs may adversely affect the autonomic tone by reducing HRV, with a potential pro-arrhythmic effect as a consequence. Drugs that may reduce HRV should be avoided in patients with CAN: only resting tachycardia associated with CAN can be treated with cardioselective β blockers [1, 22].

The Diabetes Control and Complications Trial (DCCT) found that intensive insulin treatment in type 1 diabetic patients reduced the incidence of CAN by 53% compared to conventional therapy [23]. The effect on CAN of intensive glycemic

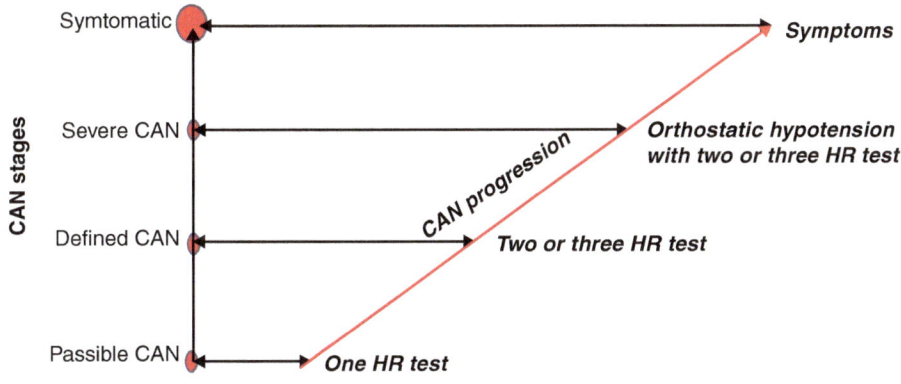

Fig. 11.1 Stages of cardiovascular autonomic neuropathy

control in patients with T2DM is still unclear. The Steno-2 trial demonstrated that intensive multifactorial treatment, including behavior modification and intensive therapy targeting hyperglycemia and CVD risk factors, lowered progression to autonomic neuropathy in patients with T2DM, as indicated by HRV during paced breathing and orthostatic hypotension (OR 0.32, 95% CI 0.12–0.78); these benefits were sustained at the 2-year follow-up [13]. Ziegler et al. reported that alpha lipoic acid improves autonomic function and is one of the few drugs endorsed by the Toronto Consensus for treating CAN [24].

Diabetes Mellitus and Orthostatic Hypotension

Orthostatic hypotension (OH) is defined as a reduction in systolic blood pressure (SBP) >20 mmHg or diastolic blood pressure (DBP) >10 mmHg in response to a postural change from supine to standing within 3 minutes. Orthostatic symptoms such as light-headedness, dizziness, blurred vision or fainting, or pain in the neck or shoulder when standing have been found to be present in 4–18% patients with diabetes mellitus (DM). OH is associated with a worse prognosis than cardiovagal neuropathy, particularly in elderly patients with DM, and may indicate an increased risk of mortality and cardiovascular events [1, 2].

Prevalence

The prevalence of OH is higher in patients with DM than those without, and both DM and OH are strong predictors of mortality and cardiovascular events. A meta-analysis of 21 studies found the prevalence of OH in patients with DM to range from 7.0% to 64.4%, with a pooled prevalence of 24%. The meta-analysis organized the diabetic patient population into subgroups according to type of DM, methodological quality score, sample size, country, and definition of OH. The pooled prevalence of OH in the subgroups ranged from 19% to 29%, and heterogeneity was high: the I^2 value ranged from 78.7% to 98.4% [5]. The analysis attributed differences in the prevalence of OH to two main reasons:

(a) The cutoff point used to determine OH based on the drop in systolic blood pressure (SBP) in response to a postural change from supine to standing was set at >20 or 30 mmHg, with diastolic blood pressure (DBP) being >10 mmHg.
(b) In elderly patients with DM, BP was measured while seated rather than standing, as the subjects are often unable to stand up.

Pathomechanism

Although OH is a sign of severe CAN, it may also occur due to reduced intravascular volume, baroreceptor reflex, and inadequate sympathetic and cardiovascular responses which may lead to reduced cardiac output. OH can also develop as a result of efferent sympathetic vasomotor denervation leading to a defective reflex arc; this culminates in an inadequate HR response and a decrease in peripheral vascular resistance when a patient stands [18, 19]. Other factors such as postprandial blood pooling, the hypotensive role of insulin, treatment by diuretics, and vasodilators or tricyclic antidepressants can accelerate the symptoms of OH. OH is associated with a worse prognosis than cardiovagal neuropathy [1, 20].

DM patients with OH have been found to demonstrate more advanced arterial stiffness than DM patients without OH, suggesting that arterial stiffness is involved in the regulation of postural BP in patients with DM, independent of cardiac autonomic activity. Poor glycemic control, as indicated by high HbA1c levels and insulin use, is associated with a higher prevalence of the later stages of cardiovascular autonomic neuropathy, when OH is more likely to occur [21].

Risk Factors

In the diabetic population, risk factors associated with OH include female sex, higher SBP, HbA1c, current smoking, and older age, as well as comorbidities such as hypertension, heart and kidney failure, and the use of β-blockers, α-blockers, and insulin [5, 7]. However, the risk factors in each study were not uniform. A meta-analysis by Zhou et al. identified seven risk factors from nine studies which were eligible for exploratory analysis: age, sex, HbA1c, BMI, supine SBP, hypertension, and diabetic nephropathy. In addition, a high level of glycosylated hemoglobin A (HbA1c), hypertension, and diabetic nephropathy were found to significantly increase the risk of OH in DM. OH was not found to have any significant relationship with age, sex, BMI or supine SBP. A high HbA1c level can affect vascular elasticity and reduce extravascular volume due to osmotic diuresis. Furthermore, poor glycemic control may cause decreased vasodilation and reduce the myo-inositol content, thus inducing OH caused by diminished blood flow in nerve fibers. Hypertension can decrease carotid sinus baroreflex and β-adrenergic sensitivity, and impair arterial elasticity and myocardial compliance [5].

The ACCORD BP (Action to Control Cardiovascular Risk in Diabetes Blood Pressure) trial randomly assigned 4733 patients with diabetes, ranging in age from 40 to 79 years (mean 62.1 years), to intensive therapy that targeted SBP of <120 mmHg, or to standard therapy that targeted SBP of <140 mmHg. Orthostatic blood pressure measurements in the ACCORD BP trial were made at three time points: baseline (1321 individuals), at 12 months (2625 individuals), and at 48 months (3702 individuals). The prevalence of OH was found to be 17.8% at baseline, 10.4% at 12 months, 12.8% at 48 months, and 20% at one or more of the three time points. It was found that female sex, being Caucasian, current smoking, higher baseline systolic BP and hemoglobin A1c, and the use of alpha-blockers, beta-blockers or insulin were independent risk factors associated with OH. A noteworthy difference between these findings and those of prior studies was that the prevalence of OH was not found to increase with age: epidemiologic studies typically indicate a low prevalence of OH in younger persons and a substantially greater one in older subjects [7], which may well be secondary to age-associated autonomic dysfunction. The absence of any such relationship between OH and age may be due to a combination of the higher prevalence of autonomic dysfunction in the ACCORD cohort with long-standing DM type 2 and the fact that 80 years is the upper age cutoff for trial eligibility. Furthermore the most noteworthy finding in the ACCORD BP trial is the lack of significant difference in OH prevalence, incidence or resolution between the aggressive (SBP <120 mmHg) versus standard (SBP <140 mmHg) blood pressure treatment groups at all time points. Surprisingly, the hypertensive diabetic patients treated to an SBP goal of <120 mmHg tended to display a decreased incidence of OH [7].

The Youth Cohort Study included 1646 subjects with type 1 diabetes (age 18 ± 4 years, diabetes duration 8 ± 2 years, HbA1c $9.1 \pm 1.9\%$, 76% non-Hispanic White subjects) and 252 with type 2 diabetes (age 22 ± 4 years, diabetes duration 8 ± 2 years, HbA1c $9.2 \pm 3.0\%$, 45% non-Hispanic Black subjects). CAN was correlated with poor long-term glycemic control, high blood pressure, and elevated triglyceride levels in subjects with type 1 diabetes, and with elevated triglycerides and increased urinary albumin excretion in the patients with type 2 diabetes. The Cardiovascular Autonomic Neuropathy Subcommittee of the Toronto Consensus Panel on Diabetic Neuropathy recommend CAN (including OH) screening to all asymptomatic type 2 diabetic patients at diagnosis and all type 1 diabetic patients after 5 years of disease, in particular those at greater risk of CAN because of a history of poor glycemic control (hemoglobin A1c >7%), the presence of one major cardiovascular risk factor, or the presence of macro- or microangiopathic complications [8].

Prognosis

The prognosis of OH in DM is associated with higher risk of total mortality and cardiovascular events. Fleg et al. demonstrated that the occurrence of OH was an independent marker of total mortality, heart failure death, or hospitalization; they also found OH to be associated with 1.62× greater all-cause mortality and 1.85× greater chance of death or hospitalization due to heart failure, but not with nonfatal myocardial infarction, stroke, cardiovascular death, or their composite [7]. In a 10-year follow-up retrospective study, Gaspar et al. found the 10-year mortality rate to be higher in diabetic patients with OH. A prospective cohort study by Wijkman et al. showed that OH in DM was not significantly associated with the risk of a combined end-point: the first nonfatal or fatal event of hospitalization for acute MI, stroke, or cardiovascular mortality [12].

In the ACCORD study, OH was associated with increased risk of total death (HR = 1.61; 95%CI 1.11–2.36) and death or hospitalization for heart failure (HR = 1.85; 95%CI 1.17–2.93). OH was found to be common in patients with type 2 diabetes and hypertension and not associated with intensive versus standard BP treatment goals. A post hoc analysis of data from ACCORD BP showed that the primary cardiovascular disease outcome was 26% lower in individuals randomized to aggressive therapy (SBP <120 mmHg) and standard glycaemia goals than in those randomized to standard therapy (SBP <140 mmHg) and standard glycaemia goals. In diabetic autonomic neuropathy, the higher mortality associated with OH may be attributed to the development of left ventricular hypertrophy. In addition, an SBP of <120 mmHg in ACCORD BP was associated with a 39% reduced risk of electrocardiographic left ventricular hypertrophy. A reduction of left ventricular hypertrophy has been found to reduce cardiovascular events [7].

Treatment

When treating symptomatic OH, especially in elderly patients with diabetes, the initial approach should consider the exclusion of drugs exacerbating OH, correction of intravascular volume, and other nonpharmacological measures. Nonpharmacological interventions include increasing water consumption, avoiding sudden changes in body posture, reducing physical maneuvers that increase intra-abdominal and intra-thoracic pressure, the use of stockings of the lower extremities, and eating smaller and more frequent meals. Pharmacotherapy should include midodrine or fludrocortisone as monotherapy, or a combination of the two in non-responders. Midodrine is the only medication approved by the Food and Drug Administration for the treatment of symptomatic OH and is now under reconsideration. It is not yet known whether pharmacological treatment of OH will alter mortality rates.

Diabetes Mellitus and Postprandial Hypotension

Postprandial hypotension (PPH) is defined as a reduction in systolic blood pressure (SBP) >20 mmHg following a meal. Postprandial hypotension is a common cause of falls in older persons and diabetics with autonomic neuropathy [25]. The pathophysiology of PPH is multifactorial and the exact mechanisms remain largely unknown.

Prevalence

The prevalence of PPH have been found to be present in up to 44% of patients with recently diagnosed uncomplicated type 2 diabetes [26]. In patients with a T2DM-duration of over 5 years without clinical signs of autonomic neuropathy, PPH occurred in up to 70% of the patients after a mixed meal [38]. Smits et al. showed that postprandial hypotension was observed in two control subjects (13.3%), no metabolic syndrome subjects, and four type 2 diabetes patients (26.7%). In type 2 diabetes patients, DBP dropped up to −10.7 ± 4, 5% following a high-fat mixed meal. Moreover this study showed drop in LF/HF ratio in patients with type 2 diabetes, suggesting an increase in parasympathetic activity. Data showed that increased amounts of insulin resistance and HbA1c are associated with a postprandial decrease in BP and systemic vascular resistance (SVR) [39, 41].

Pathomechanism

The mechanisms mediating postprandial hypotension remain unclear; however, a number of factors have been implicated, including the release of gastrointestinal hormones (GLP-1, GLP-2, and GIP), meal composition, gastric emptying rate, and impaired sympathetic nervous activity. GLP-1 is known to be involved in the atrial secretion of atrial natriuretic peptide, which leads to vasodilation and natriuresis. In the postprandial state, BP may drop due to vasodilation by increased perfusion of the splanchnic vascular bed, in support of digestion and nutrient absorption. In order to maintain postprandial BP, compensatory increases in HR, stroke volume, and thus cardiac output occur [40]. Dysfunction of the autonomic nervous system may hamper these compensatory changes in elderly subjects and patients with long-standing type 2 diabetes. The mechanisms underlying PPH in patients with uncomplicated type 2 diabetes remain unstudied [39].

Diabetes Mellitus and Carotid Sinus Hypersensitivity

Carotid sinus hypersensitivity (CSH) is a well-described cause of syncope, resulting in bradycardia, exaggerated hypotension, profound bradycardia, or asystolic pauses in response to carotid sinus stimulation. Cardiovascular risk factors such as increasing age and type 2 diabetes have been associated with an increased prevalence of CSH [27]. The European Society of Cardiology defined this condition as asystole lasting for at least 3 seconds, or a drop in systolic blood pressure (BP) of at least 50 mmHg, provoked by 5–10 seconds of carotid sinus massage (CSM). CSH is an important and frequently overlooked explanation for fainting-related falls in older adults with diabetes [29].

Prevalence

CSH is a disease of older people, with a prevalence of between 25% and 48% in patients referred to hospital for unexplained syncope, falls or dizziness. The incidence increases with age with an average age of onset at 61 to 74 years. Men are more affected than women (2:1) [29]. The prevalence of vasodepressive carotid sinus hypersensitivity (V-CSM) in older adults with T2DM was $13 \pm 10\%$ if the required decrease in SBP was defined as 50 mmHg, and $58 \pm 15\%$ if V-CSM was defined as a decrease in SBP of 30 mmHg [30]. Schwartz et al. in the prospective cohort study that included 9249 women ≥67 years of age showed that women with diabetes had higher age-specific rates of falls than women without diabetes. Women with diabetes who were not using insulin had a 68% greater risk of falling more than once a year compared with women without diabetes. Women using insulin had more than double the risk of falling more than once a year than women without diabetes [34].

Pathomechanism

The carotid sinus is an important regulator of blood pressure, and initiates the arterial baroreflex. Three types of CSH have been described: cardioinhibitory type, vasodepressor type, and mixed type. Vasodepressive carotid sinus hypersensitivity represents a common intractable condition in older adults with type 2 diabetes [32]. If the carotid sinus is hypersensitive, a patient can respond to a normal upward swing in blood pressure with a temporary stopping of the heart and an inappropriate dilatation of the vasculature. The most commonly accepted hypothesis behind CSH is that central upregulation of the arterial baroreflex occurs in response to reduced afferent input from the carotid sinus due to arterial stiffenin. This hypersensitive response leads to decreased blood flow to the brain, precipitating unexplained falls and faints [31]. CSH may be a part of a generalized autonomic disorder associated with autonomic dysregulation. Data have been reported on neuronal degeneration with accumulation of hyperphosphorylated tau or alpha-synuclein in neurones in medulla, leading to impairment of central regulation of baroreflex responses and predispose elderly patients with diabetes to CSH. Parasympathetic damage occurs earlier in the course of diabetes than extracardiac sympathetic activity. An overreaction of the carotid sinus baroreceptors stimulated by sympathetic activity may cause CSH in diabetes patients [28].

Prognosis

CSH is associated with an increased risk of falls, drop attacks, bodily injuries, and fractures in elderly patients. Brignole et al. showed that the mortality rate after 5 years was 34% in the CSH group, compared with 27% in the control group. The mortality rate in the CSH group was not influenced by CSH subtype. Similar findings were reported by Sutton et al.; the 5-year mortality rate was 36% [33].

Treatment

V-CSH has no recognized pharmacological treatment. Pacemakers have been shown to be effective in older adults with pure cardioinhibitory CSH, but have a 62% failure rate in older adults with mixed CSH. Pacemakers have no impact at all on pure V-CSH and are not recommended in this population [30].

Diabetes Mellitus and Post- exercise Hypotension

Post-exercise hypotension (PEH) is a prolonged reduction in blood pressure (BP) after a single exercise bout to values lower than pre-exercise resting [35].

Type 2 diabetes mellitus (DM2) has been associated with obesity, dyslipidemia, endothelial dysfunction, and arterial hypertension (AH). Chronic hyperglycemia and hyperinsulinemia induce vascular dysfunction leading to an increased arterial resistance and AH. Since DM2 is associated with endothelial disturbance, it is important to analyze if PEH may be presented by DM2 individuals. The Lima et al. study suggests that the exercise intensity has an important role on PEH induction and blood pressure control for DM2. Resistance exercise (RE) performed at an intensity of 70% of one repetition maximum strength test promoted PEH in T2D individuals. The exercise at 110% anaerobic threshold (AT) promoted significant PEH of mean arterial pressure (MAP). Furthermore, MAP levels during the post-exercise recovery from the exercise at 110% AT were below those of the control session [36]. PEH has been widely described for healthy and hypertensive individuals, there is a lack in the literature of studies analyzing PEH on diabetes [37].

Key Points

- Elderly patients with long-standing type 2 diabetes and autonomic neuropathy had high prevalence of PPH.
- Risk factors associated with hypotensive syndrome include female sex, higher SBP, HbA1c, current smoking, older age, as well as comorbidities such as hypertension, cardiac failure, and kidney failure, and the use of β-blockers, α-blockers, and insulin.
- All type 2 diabetic patients should be screened for OH at diagnosis, and all type 1 diabetic patients after 5 years of disease, particularly those at greater risk of OH due to a history of poor glycemic control (hemoglobin A1c >7%), the presence of one major cardiovascular risk factor or the presence of macro or microangiopathic complications.
- Treatment of elevated SBP to an intensive target of 120 mmHg does not increase the risk of OH; furthermore, SBP <120 mm Hg was associated with a 39% reduced risk of electrocardiographic left ventricular hypertrophy, resulting in a reduction of cardiovascular events.

References

1. Vinik AI, Ziegler D. Diabetic cardiovascular autonomic neuropathy. Circulation. 2007;115(3):387–97.
2. Kempler P, Tesfaye S, Chaturvedi N, et al. Blood pressure response to standing in the diagnosis of autonomic neuropathy: the EURODIAB IDDM Complications Study. Arch Physiol Biochem. 2001;109:215–22.
3. Spallone V, Ziegler D, Freeman R, et al. Cardiovascular autonomic neuropathy in diabetes: clinical impact, assessment, diagnosis, and management. Diabetes Metab Res Rev. 2011;27(7):639–53.

4. Freeman R. Diabetic autonomic neuropathy. Handb Clin Neurol. 2014;126:63–79.
5. Zhou Y, Ke S-J, Qiu X-P, et al. Prevalence, risk factors and prognosis of orthostatic hypotension in diabetic patients. A systematic review and meta-analysis. Medicine. 2017;96(36):e8004.
6. Fisher VL, Tahrani AA. Cardiac autonomic neuropathy in patients with diabetes mellitus: current perspectives. Diabetes Metab Syndr Obes. 2017;10:419–34.
7. Fleg JL, Evans GW, Margolis KL, Barzilay J, Basile JN, Bigger JT, Cutler JA, Grimm R, Pedley C, Peterson K, Pop-Busui R, Sperl-Hillen J, Cushman WC. Orthostatic hypotension in the ACCORD (Action to Control Cardiovascular Risk in Diabetes) blood pressure trial: prevalence, incidence, and prognostic significance. Hypertension. 2016;68:888–95.
8. Jaiswal M, Divers J, Urbina EM, et al. Cardiovascular autonomic neuropathy in adolescents and young adults with type 1 and type 2 diabetes: the SEARCH for Diabetes in Youth Cohort Study. Pediatr Diabetes. 2018;19:680–9.
9. Maser RE, Mitchell BD, Vinik AI, Freeman R. The association between cardiovascular autonomic neuropathy and mortality in individuals with diabetes: a meta-analysis. Diabetes Care. 2003;26(6):1895–901.
10. Ziegler D, Zentai CP, Perz S, et al. Prediction of mortality using measures of cardiac autonomic dysfunction in the diabetic and nondiabetic population: the MONICA/KORA Augsburg Cohort Study. Diabetes Care. 2008;31:556–61.
11. Veglio M, Chinaglia A, Cavallo-Perin P. QT interval, cardiovascular risk factors and risk of death in diabetes. J Endocrinol Investig. 2004;27:175–81.
12. Wijkman M, Lanne T, Ostgren CJ, et al. Diastolic orthostatic hypertension and cardiovascular prognosis in type 2 diabetes: a prospective cohort study. Cardiovasc Diabetol. 2016;15:83.
13. Gæde P, Oellgaard J, Carstensen B, et al. Years of life gained by multifactorial intervention in patients with type 2 diabetes mellitus and microalbuminuria: 21 years follow-up on the Steno-2 randomised trial. Diabetologia. 2016;59(11):2298–307.
14. Shah MS, Brownlee M. Molecular and cellular mechanisms of cardiovascular disorders in diabetes. Circ Res. 2016;118(11):1808–29.
15. Gibbons C, Centi J, Vernino S, Freeman R. Autoimmune autonomic ganglionopathy with reversible cognitive impairment. Arch Neurol. 2012;69(4):461–6.
16. Vinik AI, Erbas T, Casellini CM. Diabetic cardiac autonomic neuropathy, inflammation and cardiovascular disease. J Diabet Investig. 2013;4(1):4–18. https://doi.org/10.1111/jdi.12042.
17. Tahrani AA, Ali A, Raymond NT, et al. Obstructive sleep apnea and diabetic neuropathy: a novel association in patients with type 2 diabetes. Am J Respir Crit Care Med. 2012;186(5):434–41.
18. Low PA, Benrud-Larson LM, Sletten DM, et al. Autonomic symptoms and diabetic neuropathy: a population-based study. Diabetes Care. 2004;27(12):2942–7.
19. Low PA, Walsh JC, Huang CY, McLeod JG. The sympathetic nervous system in diabetic neuropathy. A clinical and pathological study. Brain. 1975;98:341–56.
20. Kuehl M, Stevens MJ. Cardiovascular autonomic neuropathies as complications of diabetes mellitus. Nat Rev Endocrinol. 2012;8(7):405–16.
21. Kobayashi Y, Fujikawa T, Kobayashi H, et al. Relationship between arterial stiffness and blood pressure drop during the sit-to-stand test in patients with diabetes mellitus. J Atheroscler Thromb. 2017;24(2):147–56.
22. Aronson D. Pharmacologic modulation of autonomic tone: implications for the diabetic patient. Diabetologia. 1997;40:476–81.
23. Anonymous. Assessment: clinical autonomic testing report of the therapeutics and technology assessment Subcommittee of the American Academy of Neurology. Neurology. 1996;46:873–80.
24. Pop-Busui R, Evans GW, Gerstein HC, et al. Effects of cardiac autonomic dysfunction on mortality risk in the Action to Control Cardiovascular Risk in Diabetes (ACCORD) trial. Diabetes Care. 2010;33(7):1578–84.
25. Jansen RW, Lipsitz LA. Postprandial hypotension: epidemiology, pathophysiology, and clinical management. Ann Intern Med. 1995;122:286–95.
26. Jones KL, Tonkin A, Horowitz M, Wishart JM, Carney BI, Guha S, et al. Rate of gastric emptying is a determinant of postprandial hypotension in non-insulin-dependent diabetes mellitus. Clin Sci. 1998;94:65–70.

27. Healey J, Connolly SJ, Morillo CA. The management of patients with carotid sinus syndrome: is pacing the answer? Clin Auton Res. 2004;14:80–6.
28. Ziegler D. Cardiovascular autonomic neuropathy: clinical manifestations and measurement. Diabetes Rev. 1999;7:300–15.
29. Allcock LM, O'shea D. Diagnostic yield and development of a neurocardiovascular investigation unit for older adults in a district hospital. J Gerontol A Biol Sci Med Sci. 2000;55:458–62.
30. Madden KM, et al. Aerobic training in older adults with type 2 diabetes and vasodepressive carotid sinus hypersensitivity. Aging Clin Exp Res. 2013;25(6):651–7.
31. O'Mahony D. Pathophysiology of carotid sinus hypersensitivity in elderly patients. Lancet. 1995;346:950–2.
32. Graux P, Guymar Y, Carliez R, Lemaire N, Dutoit A, Croccel L. Secondary carotid sinus syndrome. In: Blanc JJ, Benditt DG, Sutton R, editors. Neurally mediated Syncope. Armonk: Futura Publishing Co Inc; 1996. p. 145–51.
33. Hampton JL, Brayne C, Bradley M, Kenny RA. Mortality in carotid sinus hypersensitivity: a cohort study. BMJ. 2011;1:1–5.
34. Schwartz AV, et al. Older women with diabetes have a higher risk of falls: a prospective study. Diabetes Care. 2002;25:1749–54.
35. Pescatello LS, Guidry MA, Blanchard BE, et al. Exercise intensity alters postexercise hypotension. J Hypertens. 2004;22:1881–8.
36. Lima LCJ, et al. Hypotensive effects of exercise performed around an aerobic threshold in type 2 diabetic patients. Diabetes Res Clin Pract. 2008;81(2):216–22.
37. Quinn TJ. Twenty-four hour ambulatory blood pressure responses following acute exercise: impact of exercise intensity. J Hum Hypertens. 2000;14:547–53.
38. Tanakaya M, Takahashi N, Takeuchi K, Katayama Y, Yumoto A, Kohno K, et al. Postprandial hypotension due to a lack of sympathetic compensation in patients with diabetes mellitus. Acta Med Okayama. 2007;61:191–7.
39. Smits MM, et al. Uncomplicated human type 2 diabetes is associated with meal-induced blood pressure lowering and cardiac output increase. Diabetes Res Clin Pract. 2014 Dec;106(3):617–26.
40. Scott EM, Greenwood JP, Vacca G, Stoker JB, Gilbey SG, Mary DA. Carbohydrate ingestion, with transient endogenous insulinaemia, produces both sympathetic activation and vasodilatation in normal humans. Clin Sci (Lond). 2002;102:523–9.
41. Ryan JP, Sheu LK, Verstynen TD, Onyewuenyi IC, Gianaros PJ. Cerebral blood flow links insulin resistance and baroreflex sensitivity. PLoS One. 2013;8:e83288.

Hypotensive Syndromes and Heart Failure

12

Kannayiram Alagiakrishnan, Darren Mah, and Ali Ahmed

Introduction

The prevalence of heart failure (HF) increases with age, and the majority of patients are older adults [1]. It is part of the end-stage presentation of many cardiac conditions including cardiomyopathies and hypertensive, ischemic, arrhythmic, and valvular heart disease. Despite numerous available medical and device therapies, HF is a source of great morbidity leading to decreased functional activity and quality of life. Hypotensive syndromes are a disorder with a cardiovascular and autonomic etiology. This chapter discusses the relationship between hypotensive syndromes and HF.

Role of Autonomic Dysfunction in HF and Its Possible Association with Different Hypotensive Syndromes

Autonomic dysfunction often leads to different hypotensive syndromes. Heart failure is a complex disease, often with comorbid autonomic nervous system (ANS) dysfunction [2]. The arterial baroreceptor system contributes to the neural regulation of the cardiovascular system. The ANS regulates heart rate and blood pressure.

K. Alagiakrishnan
Division of Geriatric Medicine, University of Alberta, Edmonton, AB, Canada

D. Mah
University of Alberta, Edmonton, AB, Canada

A. Ahmed (✉)
Washington DC VA Medical Center and George Washington University and Georgetown University, Washington, DC, USA
e-mail: Ali.Ahmed@va.gov

© Springer Nature Switzerland AG 2020
K. Alagiakrishnan, M. Banach (eds.), *Hypotensive Syndromes in Geriatric Patients*, https://doi.org/10.1007/978-3-030-30332-7_12

117

Baroreceptors monitor changes in blood pressure to maintain adequate cerebral perfusion through stretch receptors in the carotid sinuses and aortic arch. A decrease in systemic blood pressure results in deactivation of baroreceptors with a subsequent enhancement of sympathetic activity and vagal inhibition, leading to tachycardia and increased cardiac contractility, vascular resistance, and venous return [3]. In HF, the ANS plays a role in maintaining cardiovascular homeostasis [4]. Activation of the sympathetic nervous activity and parasympathetic withdrawal causes myocardial damage in HF patients [5].

Increased sympathetic nervous system (SNS) activity is seen in both types of HF, HF with preserved ejection fraction and HF with reduced ejection fraction. This increased SNS activity maintains cardiac output initially via positive inotropic and chronotropic effects. Chronic activation of the SNS and withdrawal of parasympathetic nervous system (PSNS) input may lead to progressive myocardial dysfunction in HF. As HF progresses, inhibitory input from arterial and cardiopulmonary receptors decreases and excitatory input increases [6–11]. With increased SNS activation comes increased apoptosis, abnormal calcium handling, and increased interstitial fibrosis, leading to myocardial dysfunction [12–14].

Autonomic testing evaluates the parasympathetic and sympathetic nervous system. Autonomic system markers involve measures of heart rate (or RR interval) and blood pressure, either spontaneously or following provocations. A marked reduction of heart rate variability (HRV) is found in patients with chronic HF [15, 16]. There are numerous techniques available to assess autonomic function, but only a limited number of tests are suitable for routine clinical applications (Table 12.1) [17, 18].

Heart Rate Variability

Resting heart rate can be thought as a combination of the body's SNS and PSNS inputs to the heart. Fluctuations in resting heart rate are related to the dynamic between the body's autonomic nervous system and the heart. There are numerous ways to measure HRV. The two main categories of measurement can be described as [1] time domain (time between successive normal heart beats) and [2] frequency

Table 12.1 Selected tests of autonomic function

(a) Tests of Cardioadrenergic Function
Blood pressure response to standing
Blood pressure response to head-up tilt table testing
Blood pressure response to eating
Blood pressure response to exercise
Plasma catecholamine levels supine vs. standing
(b) Tests of Cardiovagal Function
Heart rate variability after cyclic deep breathing
Heart rate response to Valsalva maneuver
Heart rate response to standing

domain (distribution of time between successive normal heart beats). Within the frequency domain, low-frequency and high-frequency measurements may represent sympathetic activity and parasympathetic activity, respectively, and the low/high frequency ratio may be thought to reflect the balance between the two [15, 19]. Heart rate variability during and after exercise has been measured and used to assess the autonomic nervous system. The return to baseline heart rate after exercise-induced tachycardia is mediated by increased parasympathetic activity and decreased sympathetic activity [20].

(a) Simple ECG: The RR interval in a simple ECG recording varies from beat to beat mainly in response to changes in autonomic function. HRV is an estimate of these beat-to-beat variations, and it is a non-invasive approach to evaluate autonomic modulation of the heart [21]. HRV gives a quantitative measure of autonomic activity but provides a qualitative index of changes in cardiac autonomic regulation.

(b) 24-hour ECG monitoring: The RR intervals from an entire 24-hour ECG recording are often used to assess HRV. The longer recording allows more in-depth analysis of HRV. Heart rate variability can be assessed after various challenges including the Valsalva maneuver, standing and tilt-table studies, and exercise.

Baroreflex Sensitivity

Baroreflex sensitivity (BRS) is evaluated by the relationship between changes in the RR interval in response to increases or decreases in blood pressure elicited by phenylephrine or nitroglycerine respectively [22].

Measures of baroreflex function help with risk stratification, assessment of treatment effect, and prognostic evaluation in cardiovascular disease, although these techniques are presently of limited value in daily clinical practice. Non-pharmacological therapies like carotid baroreceptor stimulation, vagal nerve stimulation, spinal cord stimulation, and renal denervation may play a future role in the management of heart failure and hypotensive syndromes [23].

Hypotensive Syndromes and Their Association with HF

Orthostatic Hypotension and HF

Orthostatic hypotension (OH) is a disorder associated with different cardiovascular conditions. Although patients are generally asymptomatic or have minimal symptoms, studies have shown OH is an independent risk factor for HF. OH itself may also complicate treatment of HF.

The prevalence of OH in patients with HF varies considerably, ranging from approximately 8% in community-dwelling adults to 83% of elderly hospitalized patients [24]. In patients with HF, there are several risk factors that predispose to OH. These include severe HF, prolonged bed rest, and the number of medications used to treat HF [24].

OH in older adults is associated with coronary artery disease (CAD), a major risk factor for incident HF. OH has also been shown to directly play a role in HF development by the Rotterdam Study [25]. In the Malmo Preventive project, OH predicts incident HF in middle-aged adults. Notably, the strength of the relationship between OH and HF was somewhat attenuated when subjects with hypertension were excluded [26]. Within the Cardiovascular Health Study (CHS) cohort, Alagiakrishnan et al. showed symptomatic OH predicts incident HF [27]. Guichard et al. in the same CHS cohort showed isolated diastolic hypotension was associated with a 33% increased risk of incident HF after 12 years of follow-up (HR 1.33, 95% CI 1.10–1.61) in community-dwelling older adults [28].

In the ARIC (Atherosclerosis Risk in Communities) study, 12,363 Caucasian and African-American adults were followed for 17.5 years. OH was associated with incident HF after multivariable adjustment (HR 1.54, 95% CI 1.30–1.82), and a stronger association was identified in individuals ≤55 years old (HR 1.90, 95% CI 1.41–2.55) than in those older than 55 years (HR 1.37, 95% CI 1.12–1.69). Antihypertensive medications did not appear to play a large role in the association of OH and HF [29].

Studies that have examined the association between OH and HF have not always followed the most current OH measurement guidelines [30]. In these cases, the differences seen in prevalence and incidence could be at least partially related to inconsistency in measurement. In addition, delayed OH was not measured in some of these studies.

Mechanisms of Orthostatic Hypotension and HF

OH contributes to HF in the elderly through numerous mechanisms including increased vascular stiffness [31] and baroreflex dysfunction [32]. In younger patients, vascular disease and sub- clinical cardiac dysfunction may also play a role. Other causes can be due to strong diuresis or autonomic neuropathy, secondary to diabetes and/or Parkinson's disease. Risk factors for the development of OH in HF and vice versa are shown in Table 12.2.

Table 12.2 Risk factors of the development of orthostatic hypotension in HF and vice versa

Risk factors for the development of OH in HF	Risk factors for the development of HF in OH
Prolonged bed rest	Older age
Medication types (e.g., loop diuretics)	Hypertension
Polypharmacy	Diabetes mellitus
Autonomic neuropathy/dysfunction	
Aortic stenosis	
Arrhythmias	

Both supine and nocturnal hypertension are commonly seen with OH. These are both causal and risk factors for HF [33]. Baroreflex dysfunction and/or autonomic dysfunction are seen in patients with HF and may contribute to OH [34]. This autonomic imbalance results in adverse cardiac, vascular, and renal effects resulting in left ventricular hypertrophy, peripheral vasoconstriction, and salt and water retention.

Clinical Presentation of Orthostatic Hypotension in HF

The majority of HF subjects are asymptomatic with OH [35]. The most common symptoms, dizziness and weakness, were reported in 43% of female patients in a small study of older HF subjects with OH [36].

Management Considerations in Patients with Orthostatic Hypotension and HF

Because of the longitudinal association with the development of LVH independent of hypertension, it is important to detect OH in HF populations [37].

Bed rest can cause or aggravate OH in HF subjects [38].

One study reported that lower limb compression bandages prevented OH in 43% of patients; however, there was no significant amelioration of OH-related symptoms [39].

In one study, thiazide diuretics were reported to cause less postural hypotension than loop diuretics [40]. However, another study did not find an association between oral furosemide therapy and OH in acute decompensated HF [41].

HF is a relative contraindication to fludrocortisone. Recent study affirms the avoidance of fludrocortisone in patients with HF and OH, because of the increased risk of all-cause hospitalization when compared to midodrine therapy [42]. Another study reported losartan 50 mg at night time can also decrease supine hypertension without worsening orthostatic hypotension commonly seen in the early morning hours [43].

Cardiac resynchronization therapy can be considered if HF worsens OH [41, 44]. Another therapy that can be considered is baroreflex activation therapy, if available [45]. It involves electrical stimulation of the carotid baroreceptors via an implanted device resembling a cardiac pacemaker. In animal and human studies, correction of baroreceptor dysfunction using bionic baroreceptors may both improve OH and serve as potential therapy for HF [46–48].

To reduce the effects of night-time hypertension seen with OH, the head of the bed can be tilted to 30–45 degrees to reduce supine hypertension and nocturnal supine diuresis which can worsen OH upon awakening [49].

Postprandial Hypotension and HF

In a small study by Vankraaij et al., 55% of HF subjects with preserved ejection fraction were shown to have postprandial hypotension (PPH). In this study, after stopping furosemide therapy, the postprandial blood pressure decline diminished significantly. A mechanism that may be responsible for this change is that reduced intravascular volume from diuresis leads to an insufficient postprandial increase in cardiac output, exacerbating the postprandial blood pressure drop [50].

In one nursing home study, 36% of subjects had PPH, and treatment with vasodilators was associated with a more severe postprandial decline in systolic blood pressure [51]. Another study by Aronow et al. found PPH was present in 24% of nursing home subjects. PPH was significantly more common in residents treated with angiotensin-converting enzyme inhibitors, calcium channel blockers, diuretics, nitrates, digoxin, and psychotropic drugs than in residents not treated with these drugs. With more of these medications, a greater decline in postprandial systolic BP was found [52]. Chronic use of these medications in cardiovascular conditions like HF may contribute to PPH.

Carotid Sinus Hypersensitivity, Vasovagal Syncope, and HF

Carotid sinus hypersensitivity (CSH) and vasovagal syncope (VVS) are commonly seen in patients with HF and play a role in the syncope and sudden cardiac death in HF subjects. McDonald et al. showed that 9.4% of patients with HF had CSH. In the vasodepressive type of CSH, significant drops in blood pressure can occur, leading to syncope and falls [53]. Syncope is a sudden, temporary, and self-terminating loss of consciousness, often due to decreased cerebral perfusion secondary to a fall in systemic arterial pressure. CSH and VVS are common causes of neurally medicated syncope [54].

Isolated VVS should be distinguished from other forms of syncope that start in old age and which are often associated with cardiovascular, neurological, and other autonomic disturbances such as CSH and PPH. VVS can also result from general autonomic system pathology. Impaired venoconstriction (secondary to a diminished increase in peripheral resistance) and baroreflex function can lead to syncope [55, 56].

In patients with dilated cardiomyopathy who develop syncope, approximately two-thirds of cases are attributable to cardiac (arrhythmias, conduction and valvular disorders, OH) and neurological causes. However, in up to one-third of subjects, the etiology remains unidentified; potentially the above-mentioned conditions play a role in these patients [57]. Middlekauff et al. showed that syncope in HF confers a high risk for sudden death regardless of its etiology [58].

Post-exercise Hypotension and HF

Post-exercise hypotension (PEH) is a sustained reduction in systolic and/or diastolic blood pressure following exercise. Commonly, it is caused by dynamic exercise using large muscles (e.g., walking, running, cycling, and swimming), performed at intensities between 40% and 70% of maximal oxygen consumption, and continued to the point of exhaustion. On average, the maximum reductions in systolic and diastolic BP are 18–20 and 7–9 mmHg, respectively, for patients with hypertension and 8–10 and 3–5 mmHg, respectively, for those who are normotensive. Depending on the individual, PEH can persist for anywhere from 2 to 13 hours. Patients with hypertension generally have more prolonged PEH [59, 60].

Possible mechanisms mediating PEH in HF include decreased stroke volume, cardiac output, limb vascular resistance, total peripheral resistance, and muscle sympathetic discharge. Some of these changes in resistance may be explained by sustained post-exercise vasodilation.

Post-exercise hypotension can occur in patients with coronary artery disease (CAD). Approximately 8% of patients with CAD undergoing exercise testing experience a hypotensive response, and nearly 50% of these will have three-vessel or left main disease. In persons with CAD, PEH is likely due to activation of mechanoreceptors in ischemic conditions. In those who have known ischemia or left ventricular dysfunction and also experience PEH, the risk of death or MI is significantly increased during exercise. However, PEH leading to a systolic blood pressure below its resting value may be more important as a risk factor [61]. PEH has also been associated with a reduction in cardiac output [62] and altered cardiac autonomic modulation [63].

Studies recommend exercise as part of the management strategy for patients with HF [64, 65]. According to the 2013 American College of Cardiology Foundation/American Heart Association Guideline for the Management of Heart Failure Exercise Treatment (or Regular Physical Activity) is recommended as safe and effective for patients with HF who are able to participate to improve functional status (a Class I recommendation based on level of evidence A) [66]. However, exercise should be moderate and as tolerated for, because as described previously aerobic exercise can produce PEH [59, 67]. PEH is also seen in younger subjects with dilated cardiomyopathy, as evidenced by sustained calf and systemic vasodilation compared to healthy controls [68]. Advancing age in HF can also be detrimental to cardiac output due to modifications in structure and function of the cardiac muscle cells as seen in HF [69].

In autonomic failure, supine exercise lowers blood pressure and worsens postural hypotension. In these same patients, food and exercise in combination may produce a cumulative blood pressure lowering effect due to unopposed simultaneous splanchnic and skeletal muscle dilation due to lack of corrective cardiovascular reflexes [70].

Nocturnal Hypotension and HF

Studies showing the relationship between nocturnal hypotension and HF are scarce. Patients with severe HF often have altered baroreceptor and autonomic function, which may negatively influence night-time blood pressure patterns [71]. A small study by Rodrigues et al. showed a larger nocturnal BP drop was associated with more left ventricular hypertrophy [72].

Conclusions

Directly and indirectly, hypotensive syndromes can play a role in the development of HF as well as increase complications in those with HF. Ultimately, these syndromes and HF are tightly linked with common risk factors and a high shared incidence/prevalence. Pharmacological modulation of ANS may be cautiously considered in the management of hypotensive syndromes in HF when symptoms adversely affect quality of life. Presently, there is a need for future studies to understand the many unanswered questions surrounding these conditions, including ideal prevention, screening, and management.

References

1. Barker WH, Mullooly JP, Getchell W. Changing incidence and survival for heart failure in a well-defined older population, 1970–1974 and 1990–1994. Circulation. 2006;113:799–805.
2. Kishi T. Heart failure as an autonomic nervous system dysfunction. J Cardiol. 2012;59:117–22.
3. Kirchheim HR. Systemic arterial baroreceptor reflexes. Physiol Rev. 1976;56:100–77.
4. Kishi T. Heart failure as a disruption of dynamic circulatory homeostasis mediated by brain. Int Heart J. 2016;57:145–9.
5. Floras JS. Clinical aspects of sympathetic activation and parasympathetic withdrawal in heart failure. J Am Coll Cardiol. 1993;22:72A–84A.
6. Zhang DY, Anderson AS. The sympathetic nervous system and heart failure. Cardiol Clin. 2014;32(1):33–45.
7. Watson AM, Hood SG, May CN. Mechanisms of sympathetic activation in heart failure. Clin Exp Pharmacol Physiol. 2006;33:1269–74.
8. Pepper GS, Lee RW. Sympathetic activation in heart failure and its treatment with beta-blockade. Arch Intern Med. 1999;159:225–34.
9. Grassi G, Seravalle G, Quarti-Trevano F, et al. Sympathetic and baroreflex cardiovascular control in hypertension-related left ventricular dysfunction. Hypertension. 2009;53:205–9.
10. Hogg K, McMurray J. Neurohumoral pathways in heart failure with preserved systolic function. Prog Cardiovasc Dis. 2005;47:357–66.
11. Dibner-Dunlap ME, Thames MD. Control of sympathetic nerve activity by vagal mechanoreflexes is blunted in heart failure. Circulation. 1992;86:1929–34.
12. Piacentino V, Weber CR, Chen X, et al. Cellular basis of abnormal calcium transients of failing human ventricular myocytes. Circ Res. 2003;92:651–8.
13. Brouri F, Hanoun N, Mediani O, et al. Blockade of beta 1- and desensitization of beta 2-adrenoceptors reduce isoprenaline-induced cardiac fibrosis. Eur J Pharmacol. 2004;485:227–34.

14. Dunlap ME, Bibevski S, Rosenberry TL, Ernsberger P. Mechanisms of altered vagal control in heart failure: influence of muscarinic receptors and acetylcholinesterase activity. Am J Physiol Heart Circ Physiol. 2003;285:H1632–40.
15. Saul JP, Arai Y, Berger RD, et al. Assessment of autonomic regulation in chronic congestive heart failure by heart rate spectral analysis. Am J Cardiol. 1988;61:1292–9.
16. Kinugawa T, Dibner-Dunlap ME. Altered vagal and sympathetic control of heart rate in left ventricular dysfunction and heart failure. Am J Phys. 1995;268:R310–6.
17. Adamopoulos S, Piepoli M, McCance A, et al. Comparison of different methods for assessing sympathovagal balance in chronic congestive heart failure secondary to coronary artery disease. Am J Cardiol. 1992;70:1576–82.
18. Lahiri MK, Kannankeril PJ, Goldberger JJ. Assessment of autonomic function in cardiovascular disease: physiological basis and prognostic implications. J Am Coll Cardiol. 2008;51:1725–33.
19. La Rovere MT, Pinna GD, Maestri R, et al. Short-term heart rate variability strongly predicts sudden cardiac death in chronic heart failure patients. Circulation. 2003;107:565–70.
20. Piotrowicz E, Baranowski R, Piotrowska M, et al. Variable effects of physical training of heart rate variability, heart rate recovery, and heart rate turbulence in chronic heart failure. Pacing Clin Electrophysiol. 2009;32(Suppl 1):S113–5.
21. Heart rate variability. Standards of measurement, physiological interpretation, and clinical use. Task force of the European Society of Cardiology and the North American Society of Pacing and Electrophysiology. Eur Heart J. 1996;17:354–81.
22. Smyth HS, Sleight P, Pickering GW. Reflex regulation of arterial pressure during sleep in man. A quantitative method for assessing baroreflex sensitivity. Circ Res. 1969;24:109–21.
23. Chatterjee NA, Singh JP. Novel intervention therapies to modulate the autonomic tone in heart failure. JACC Heart Failure. 2015;3(10):786–802.
24. Gorelik O, Feldman L, Cohen N. Heart failure and orthostatic hypotension. Heart Fail Rev. 2016;21:529–38.
25. Verwoert GC, Mattace- Raso FU, Hofman A, et al. Orthostatic hypotension and risk of cardiovascular disease in the elderly people: the Rotterdam study. J Am Geriatr Soc. 2008;56(10):1816–20.
26. Fedorowski A, Engström G, Hedblad B, et al. Orthostatic hypotension predicts incidence of heart failure: the Malmö preventive project. Am J Hypertens. 2010;23:1209–15.
27. Alagiakrishnan K, Patel K, Desai RV, et al. Orthostatic hypotension and incident heart failure in community-dwelling older adults. J Gerontol A Biol Sci Med Sci. 2014;69:223–30.
28. Guichard JL, Desai RV, Ahmed MI, et al. Isolated diastolic hypotension and incident heart failure in older adults. Hypertension. 2011;58(5):895–901.
29. Jones CD, Loehr L, Franceschini N, et al. Orthostatic hypotension as a risk factor for incident heart failure: the Atherosclerosis Risk in Communities (ARIC) study. Hypertension. 2012;59(5):913–8.
30. Freeman R, Wieling W, Axelrod FB, et al. Consensus statement on the definition of orthostatic hypotension, neurally mediated syncope and the postural tachycardia syndrome. Clin Auton Res. 2011;21:69–72.
31. Mattace-Raso FU, van der Cammen TJ, Knetsch AM, et al. Arterial stiffness as the candidate underlying mechanism for postural blood pressure changes and orthostatic hypotension in older adults: the Rotterdam study. J Hypertens. 2006;24:339–44.
32. James MA, Potter JF. Orthostatic blood pressure changes and arterial baroreflex sensitivity in elderly subjects. Age Ageing. 1999;28:522–30.
33. Voichanski S, Grossman C, Leibowitz A, et al. Orthostatic hypotension is associated with nocturnal change in systolic blood pressure. Am J Hypertens. 2012;25:159–64.
34. Mortara A, La Rovere MT, Pinna GD, et al. Arterial baroreflex modulation of heart rate in chronic heart failure: clinical and hemodynamic correlates and prognostic implications. Circulation. 1997;96:3450–8.
35. Arbogast SD, Alshekhlee A, Hussain Z, et al. Hypotension unawareness in profound orthostatic hypotension. Am J Med. 2009;122:574–80.

36. Potocka-Plazak K, Plazak W. Orthostatic hypotension in elderly women with congestive heart failure. Aging Clin Exp Res. 2001;13:378–84.
37. Magnusson M, Holm H, Bachus E, et al. Orthostatic hypotension and cardiac changes after long-term follow-up. Am J Hypertens. 2016;29:847–52.
38. Feldstein C, Weder AB. Orthostatic hypotension: a common, serious and underrecognized problem in hospitalized patients. J Am Soc Hypertens. 2012;6:27–39.
39. Gorelik O, Almoznino-Sarafian D, Litvinov V, et al. Seating-induced postural hypotension is common in older patients with decompensated heart failure and may be prevented by lower limb compression bandaging. Gerontology. 2009;55:138–44.
40. Heseltine D, Bramble MG. Loop diuretics cause less postural hypotension than thiazide diuretics in the frail elderly. Curr Med Res Opin. 1988;11:232–5.
41. Mehagnoul-Schipper DJ, Colier WN, Hoefnagels WH, et al. Effects of furosemide versus captopril on postprandial and orthostatic blood pressure and on cerebral oxygenation in patient's ≥70 years of age with heart failure. Am J Cardiol. 2002;90:596–600.
42. Grijalva CG, Biaggioni I, Griffin MR, et al. Fludrocortisone is associated with a higher risk of all-cause hospitalizations compared with Midodrine in patients with orthostatic hypotension. J Am Heart Assoc. 2017;6(10):e006848.
43. Jones PK, Shaw BH, Raj SR. Orthostatic hypotension: managing a difficult problem. Expert Rev Cardiovasc Ther. 2015;13:1263–76.
44. Ricci F, De Caterina R, Fedorowski A. Orthostatic hypotension: epidemiology, prognosis, and treatment In a small study OH was not seen with ACE inhibitor therapy with Captopril for two weeks. J Am Coll Cardiol. 2015;66:848–60.
45. Gronda E, Seravalle G, Brambilla G, et al. Chronic baroreflex activation effects on sympathetic nerve traffic, baroreflex function, and cardiac haemodynamics in heart failure: a proof-of-concept study. Eur J Heart Fail. 2014;16:977–83.
46. Hosokawa K, Ide T, Tobushi T, et al. Bionic baroreceptor corrects postural hypotension in rats with impaired baroreceptor. Circulation. 2012;126:1278–85.
47. Sabbah HN. Baroreflex activation for the treatment of heart failure. Curr Cardiol Rep. 2012;14:326–33.
48. Georgakopoulos D, Little WC, Abraham WT, et al. Chronic baroreflex activation: a potential therapeutic approach to heart failure with preserved ejection fraction. J Card Fail. 2011;17:167–78.
49. Gibbons CH, Schmidt P, Biaggioni I, et al. The recommendations of aconsensus panel for the screening, diagnosis, and treatment of neurogenic orthostatic hypotension and associated supine hypertension. J Neurol. 2017;264:1567–82.
50. Vanjraaij DJW, Jansen RWMM, Bouwels LHR, et al. Furosemide withdrawal improves postprandial hypotension in elderly patients with heart failure and preserved left ventricular systolic function. Arch Intern Med. 1999;159:1599–605.
51. Vaitkevicius PV, Esserwein DM, Maynard AK, et al. Frequency and importance of postprandial blood pressure reduction in elderly nursing home patients. Ann Intern Med. 1991;115:865–70.
52. Aronow WS, Ahn C. Postprandial hypotension in 499 elderly persons in a long- term care facility. J Am Geriatr Soc. 1994;42:930–2.
53. Mc Donald C, Pearce MS, Newton JL, et al. Modified criteria for carotid sinus hypersensitivity are associated with increased mortality in a population-based study. Europace. 2016;18:1101–7.
54. Can I, Cytron J, Jhanjee R, et al. Neurally-mediated syncope. Minerva Med. 2009;100(4):275–92.
55. Thomson HL, Atherton JJ, Khafagi FA, et al. Failure of reflex venocostriction during exercise in patients with vasovagal syncope. Circulation. 1996;93:953–9.
56. Bechir M, Binggeli C, Corti R, et al. Dysfunctional baroreflex regulation of sympathetic nerve activity in patients with vasovagal syncope. Circulation. 2003;107:1620–5.
57. Livanis EG, Kostopoulou A, Theodorakis GN, et al. Neurocardiogenic mechanisms of unexplained syncope in idiopathic dilated cardiomyopathy. Am J Cardiol. 2007;99:558–62.
58. Middlekauff HR, Stevenson WG, Stevenson LW, et al. Syncope in advanced heart failure: high risk of sudden death regardless of origin of syncope. J Am Coll Cardiol. 1993;21:110–6.

59. Kenney MJ, Seals DR. Post exercise hypotension. Key features, mechanisms, and clinical significance. Hypertension. 1993;22(5):653–64.
60. Alagiakrishnan K, Masaki K, Schatz I, et al. Blood pressure dysregulation syndrome: the case for control throughout the circadian cycle. Geriatrics. 2001;56(3):50–6.
61. Iskandrian AS, Kegel JG, Lemlek J, et al. Mechanism of exercise-induced hypotension in coronary artery, disease. Am J Cardiol. 1992;69(19):1517–20.
62. Rondon MUPB, Alves MJNN, Braga AMFW, et al. Post exerciseblood pressure reduction in elderly hypertensive patients. J Am Col Cardiol. 2002;39(4):676–82.
63. Teixeira L, Ritti-Dias RM, Tinucci T, et al. Post-concurrent exercise hemodynamics and cardiac autonomic modulation. Eur J Appl Physiol. 2011;111(9):2069–78.
64. Antonicelli R, Spazzafumo L, Scalvini S, et al. Exercise: a "new drug" for elderly patients with chronic heart failure. Aging (Albany NY). 2016;8:860–72.
65. Kitzman DW, Brubaker PH, Morgan TM, et al. Exercise training in older patients with heart failure and preserved ejection fraction: a randomized, controlled, single-blind trial. Circ Heart Fail. 2010;3:659–67.
66. Yancy CW, Jessup M, Bozkurt B, et al. 2013 ACCF/AHA guideline for the management of heart failure: a report of the American College of Cardiology Foundation/American Heart Association Task Force on Practice Guidelines. J Am Coll Cardiol. 2013 Oct 15;62(16):e147–239.
67. Halliwill JR, Buck TM, Lacewell AN, et al. Post exercise hypotension and sustained post exercise vasodilatation: what happens after we exercise? Exp Physiol. 2013;98(1):7–18.
68. Hara K, Floras JS. After-effects of exercise on haemodynamics and muscle sympathetic nerve activity in young patients with dilated cardiomyopathy. Heart. 1996;75(6):602–8.
69. Roh J, Rhee J, Chaudhari V, et al. The role of exercise in cardiac aging: from physiology to molecular mechanisms. Circ Res. 2016;118:279–95.
70. Puvi-Rajasingham S, Smith GD, Akinola A, et al. Hypotensive and regional haemodynamic effects of exercise, fasted and after food, in human sympathetic denervation. Clin Sci (Lond). 1998;94(1):49–55.
71. Kastrup J, Wroblewski H, Sindrup J, et al. Diurnal blood pressure profile in patients with severe congestive heart failure. Dippers and non-dippers. Scand J Clin Lab Invest. 1993;53:577–83.
72. Rodrigues JCL, Amadu AM, Ghosh Dastidar A, et al. Nocturnal dipping status and left ventricular hypertrophy: a cardiac magnetic resonance imaging study. J Clin Hypertens. 2018;20(4):784–93.

Hypotensive Syndromes and Chronic Kidney Disease

13

Jolanta Malyszko and Adrian Covic

Chronic Kidney Disease and Orthostatic Hypotension

Assuming a standing position initiates a series of compensatory changes on the part of the circulation to defend blood flow to vital organs. Standing promotes the pooling of blood in the legs [1], and the adaptive circulation increases venous tone through sympathetic stimulation, coordinated in the brainstem, to limit this pooling [2]. Baroreceptors in the neck detect the decrease in arterial stretch as the cardiac output declines, and in addition to stimulating venous tone, a variable increase in heart rate is also recruited [2]. The clinical findings in normal humans subjected to this orthostatic stress in the laboratory consist of a small decline in systolic blood pressure (SBP), often a small increase in diastolic blood pressure (DBP), and a small increase in heart rate [1]. Aging, comorbidities like diabetes and Parkinson's disease, and a variety of drugs are known to exaggerate these changes [2, 3]. In some cases, the compensatory mechanisms underrespond, or are absent, resulting in a sustained fall in SBP of more than 20 mm Hg, a sustained fall in DBP of 10 mm Hg, occurring within 3 minutes of standing or a combination of these events, which are typical criteria to diagnose orthostatic intolerance [4].

Another form of OH is delayed orthostatic hypotension (DOH). In this case, BP measurement should be performed 30 minutes after verticalization. Differential diagnosis of DOH against vasovagal syndrome (VVS) is important. The syndrome accounts for approximately 40% of BP drop incidents with syncope, while OH accounts for 10% [5]. In VVS, hypotension and/or bradycardia occur in response to an exaggerated autonomic reflex. This produces a loss of consciousness lasting up

J. Malyszko (✉)
Department of Nephrology, Dialysis and Internal Medicine, Warsaw Medical University, Warszawa, Poland

A. Covic
Grigore T. Popa University of Medicine, Strada Universității, Iasi, Romania

© Springer Nature Switzerland AG 2020
K. Alagiakrishnan, M. Banach (eds.), *Hypotensive Syndromes in Geriatric Patients*, https://doi.org/10.1007/978-3-030-30332-7_13

to 20 seconds. VVS diagnosis involves a tilt test during extended verticalization (up to 45 minutes), thereby reproducing the syncope in the diagnostic laboratory. First-line treatment for patients at risk of VVS includes alpha-sympathomimetics (mido-drine, etilefrine) [6]. Both VVS and OH are associated with patient age. The risk of OH increases in patients aged ≥65 and is found in approximately 30% of the population [7]. Orthostatic hypotension (OH) results from an autonomic nervous system dysfunction and involves maladjustment of the cardiovascular system to sudden changes in body position. Elderly hypertensive patients are a special risk group for OH. Impaired cerebral circulation in this group is also a factor [8]. Causes of OH in hypertensive patients include use of some antihypertensive drugs, mainly including diuretics, ACE inhibitors, CCBs, and alpha blockers [9]. Symptoms preceding an OH incident include visual disorders, vertigo, dysarthria, and falling after vertical-ization. In addition to antihypertensive treatment, factors contributing to OH include long-term immobility, exertion unadjusted to the patient's age, and excessively large meals. A recent review of orthostatic hypertension notes that few studies have sought to characterize the prevalence of this disorder and also noted heterogeneity in the definition with increases of 5, 10, and 20 mm Hg in SBP on standing used as criteria [10]. Unlike orthostatic hypotension, there is no agreed upon threshold of SBP increase on standing to define orthostatic hypertension, as there is for ortho-static hypertension.

Prevalence of chronic kidney disease is about 10–16%, mainly in the elderly. According to K/DOQI, glomerular filtration rate (GFR) below 60 ml/min is associ-ated with the increased risk of cardiovascular morbidity and mortality. Kurtal et al. [11] reported that undiagnosed CKD is common in elderly. Moreover, in this study, about 52% of the prescribed drugs and about 65% of all prescribed drugs were those that need dose adjustment or should be avoided in renal impairment. In our study [12], we found a very high prevalence of CKD up to 61%, on the basis of estimated GFR/creatinine clearance, in elderly patients with coronary artery disease and nor-mal serum creatinine undergoing PCI. On the other hand, the most commonly CKD is associated with hypertension as kidney fiction declines, but hypotension could be also present. However, the epidemiological data are lacking.

In SPRINT, among the 8662 participants, 634 (7%) had a drop in standing BP that met criteria for orthostatic hypotension [13]. Of the participants classified as having orthostatic hypotension, 294 met the SBP criteria only, 227 met the DBP criteria only, and 113 met both the SBP and DBP criteria. In this trial, orthostatic hypotension was more frequent in older participants, women, whites, and those with CKD (eGFR <60 ml/min/1.73 m^2), albuminuria, higher BUN, lower BMI, and higher seated BP. Greater reductions in SBP on standing were associated with older age, female sex, progressively worse National Kidney Foundation eGFR stage, cur-rent smoking, a history of heart failure, atrial fibrillation, or peripheral arterial dis-ease, and several antihypertensive drug classes including beta blockers, calcium channel blockers, and combined alpha-beta blockers. Using multivariable regres-sion analysis, they observed that age > 74 years, female sex, taller height, progressively worse eGFR stage, current smoking, and several drug classes including beta blockers, calcium channel blockers, and combined alpha-beta blockers were independently associated with greater reductions in SBP on standing. In SPRINT trial, authors observed that reductions in renal function when categorized by the National Kidney Foundation eGFR staging were also associated with greater declines in SBP. Although orthostatic hypotension was found to predict incident CKD in African-Americans in the Atherosclerosis Risk in Communities Study [14], there is little known about the prevalence of orthostatic changes in SBP in patients with CKD, and their observations were novel in this regard and robust given the number of participants ($n = 2472$) with an eGFR less than 60 ml/min/1.73 m^2 in SPRINT. Finally, they observed that antidepressants and narcotics were associated with standing BP reductions. Mechanisms by which antidepressants promote an orthostatic decline in BP include negative inotropism partly through inhibition of cardiac calcium currents [15]. Narcotics may reduce BP by direct effects on the vessel [16] or through mediating histamine release [17].

Current guidelines for the treatment of HTN in patients with CKD recommend a BP goal of less than 130/80 mm Hg [18]. This BP goal has been debated because of the lack of robust clinical trial data available to support it and the potential for harm from targeting a lower BP (e.g., orthostatic hypotension) [19]. However, a review of orthostatic hypotension in the elderly suggests that RAAS blockers rarely cause orthostatic hypotension apart from their potential to cause first-dose hypotension [20]. Further research is needed to assess orthostatic hypotension as a potential ADE in other RAAS-blocking agents and in different populations of older adults with CKD. Caution should be exercised, however, by using a lower starting dose and slowly titrating to an effective dose.

Depending on symptom intensity, pharmaceutical and non-pharmaceutical treatment can be used. Non-pharmaceutical methods include recommendations for head elevation when lying down (approximately 10–12 cm) and slow and gradual verticalization, with the patient maintaining a sitting position for approximately 30 seconds before standing up fully. Other recommendations include simple exercises enhancing circulation in the lower extremities and avoiding leaning. Consumption of alcohol and large, heavy meals is inadvisable. The patient should increase their fluid intake up to approximately 2.5 l per day. If non-pharmaceutical treatment is ineffective, oral pharmaceutical treatment should be implemented. First-line treatment is dihydroergotamine, increasing vascular tone. The starting dose is 5–10 mg twice daily. Other agents used in OH treatment include sympathomimetics, such as etilefrine (Effortil®), midodrine (Gutron®), and norfenefrine (Novadral®), which increase BP by stimulating alpha- and beta-adrenergic receptors. Another class of drugs used is mineralocorticoids, for example, fludrocortisone (Cortineff®). These drugs increase BP by increasing sodium retention [21]. OH treatment is planned individually for each patient, taking into account their age, comorbidities, and overall health. Treatment success depends on appropriate pharmaceutical treatment and lifestyle changes [21].

Hypotension in Dialysis: Intradialytic Hypotension

One of the common complications of dialysis is intradialytic hypotension in 5–30% of all dialysis sessions, requiring intravenous fluid replacement in some patients, before they could safely leave the hemodialysis unit. Intradialytic hypotension may reduce the efficacy of the dialysis procedure and contributes to the excessive morbidity and mortality that is associated with hemodialysis. There is no generally accepted definition of intradialytic hypotension. Kidney Disease Outcomes Quality Initiative (KDOQI) and European Best Practice Guidelines define intradialytic hypotension as the presence of a decrease in systolic blood pressure ≥ 20 mm Hg or a decrease in mean arterial pressure by 10 mm Hg, providing the decrease in blood pressure is associated with clinical events and need for nursing interventions [22]. Sands et al. described that among 44,801 dialysis sessions in 1137 patients, 75% of subjects had at least one episode of intradialytic hypotension [23]. Santos et al. [24] reported intradialytic hypotension in more than 50% of HD sessions [25]. Differential diagnosis includes systemic infection, arrhythmias, pericardial tamponade, valvular disorders, myocardial infarction, hemolysis, hemorrhage, air embolism, and a reaction to the dialyzer membrane [24]. However, in real settings, intradialytic hypotension occurs mainly in the absence of serious medical conditions. Factors predisposing to intradialytic hypotension include rapid or excessive ultrafiltration, a rapid reduction in plasma osmolality, incorrectly low prescribed target weight, autonomic neuropathy, and diminished cardiac reserve. Other contributors to intradialytic hypotension include the intake of antihypertensive medications or the ingestion of a meal immediately before or during dialysis. Dialysate composition and its temperature may also contribute to intradialytic hypotension. It has been reported that the use of dialysate acetate, low sodium, high magnesium, and low calcium could be risk factors for hypotension [26], however, today bicarbonate dialysate is used in general practice. Dialysate temperature that is higher than body temperature has also been associated with hypotension. Other factors include also the release of adenosine during organ ischemia, the increased synthesis of endogenous vasodilators (such as nitric oxide), and inappropriately low plasma concentration of vasopressin [27]. The most common cause of intradialytic hypotension is high ultrafiltration rate, causing intravascular volume depletion beyond the level at which blood pressure can be sustained by hemodynamic compensatory mechanisms. It may happen when the rate of fluid removal by ultrafiltration (which is from the vascular space) is significantly faster than the rate of refill of the intravascular space from the interstitial space.

Normal weight without any extra fluid in your body is called "dry weight." Dry weight was previously defined as the lowest weight a patient can tolerate without the development of symptoms or hypotension [28]. In 2009, Sinha and Agarwal [29] proposed a definition that combines subjective and objective measurements. According to this definition, dry weight is defined as the lowest tolerated postdialysis weight achieved via gradual change in postdialysis weight at which there are minimal signs or symptoms of hypovolemia or hypervolemia. Excessive or rapid ultrafiltration may occur in two distinct clinical scenarios. In most common setting, in patients with large interdialytic weight gains, rapid ultrafiltration is performed to reach the prescribed target "dry weight" during dialysis session [30, 31]. In less common situation, in patients with inaccurate "dry weight" determination, without large interdialytic weight gain, excessive ultrafiltration is prescribed to reach this target [32]. It may happen with better nutrition status, better appetite, etc. after starting the renal replacement therapy and amelioration of the severe uremia. A significant reduction in increased plasma osmolality due to high level of urea/glucose during dialysis session may also contribute to intravascular volume depletion [33].

Autonomic dysfunction (dysautonomia) is reported to be present in over 50% of hemodialyzed patients; predominantly patients with long history of diabetes are particularly prone to autonomic neuropathy [34]. In the clinical setting of autonomic dysfunction, ability to mount a sufficient sympathetic response to maintain the systemic blood pressure during ultrafiltration is impaired. It could be due to downregulation of alpha-adrenergic receptors, leading to decreased the hemodynamic response to endogenous catecholamines [35] and/or a paradoxical decline in sympathetic and elevated parasympathetic nervous system activity during ultrafiltration [36, 37]. Another large group of patients prone to intradialytic hypotension are those with heart failure, cardiomegaly, or ischemic heart disease [38]. Intradialytic hypotension in this population is mainly due to poor left ventricular performance and a diminished cardiac reserve in the setting of a hemodynamic challenge [39]. It is augmented by drugs used to treat these conditions such as beta blockers, ACEi, or ARBs. It was also reported that intradialytic hypotension is more common in patients with low cardiac index and increased vascular peripheral resistance in the first 30 minutes on hemodialysis [40].

Lightheadedness, muscle cramps, nausea, vomiting, and dyspnea are typical symptoms of intradialytic hypotension. Before the drop in blood pressure is detected, some vagal symptoms, such as yawning, sighing, and hoarseness, may be observed [24]. Intradialytic hypotension is acute complication of hemodialysis and could be managed appropriately and timely. Ultrafiltration should be stopped or decreased depending on the clinical conditions, and Trendelenburg position should be introduced with patient lying flat on the back (supine position), and the feet should be placed higher than the head by 15–30°. Intravenous fluid replacement should be also instituted. Usually isotonic saline, hypertonic glucose, or 5% dextrose is used. In clinical practice, we start with 200 ml isotonic saline, if not effect is seen more saline up to 500 ml is administered. End of the HD session is to be also considered. In addition, when hypotension persists despite measures, more detailed examination for underlying cause should be performed. In particular, occult sepsis, previously unrecognized cardiac and/or pericardial disease, and gastrointestinal bleeding should be excluded. Chest and back pain and by signs of allergic reaction (urticaria, flushing, coughing, sneezing) in addition to hypotension may suggest allergic reactions to dialyzer.

In patients with recurrent episodes of intradialytic hypotension, carefully evaluation and preventive strategies should be introduced. At first "dry weight" should be reassessed. The optimal target weight is often determined empirically by trial and error ("probing"). In some patients, despite data from bioimpedance, vena cava diameter, blood volume monitoring, NT-proBNP evaluation, etc., rise in target body weight is beneficial. Regulation of the ultrafiltration rate combined with adjustment of dialysate sodium (sodium profiling) may be also considered. In patients prone to intradialytic hypotension, eating during dialysis should be avoided as peripheral vascular resistance generally drops 20–120 minutes after the ingestion of food, which may lead to a decrease in blood pressure [24]. Another issue is withdrawal of antihypertensive agents prior to dialysis, in particular taken bid or tid. In these patients, long-acting agents taken at bedtime are preferred. Limitation of sodium intake up to 1–2 g per day is recommended as excessive sodium intake results in thirst and larger extracellular volume gain that must be removed by ultrafiltration. Dialysate calcium and magnesium should be ≥ 2.25 mEq/L and ≥ 1.0 mEq/L, respectively, as low dialysate calcium and magnesium have been associated with intradialytic hypotension. Cardiac evaluation, cooling of dialysate, and an increase in dialysis time and/or frequency are to be taken into account as well. A pericardial effusion should be excluded with an echocardiogram. Cooling of dialysate could be performed either as empiric fixed reductions of dialysate temperature or isothermic dialysis. This approach has been shown to increase hemodynamic stability [41]. The 2005 Kidney Disease Outcomes Quality Initiative (KDOQI) guidelines and 2007 European Best Practice Guidelines in hemodialysis recommend the use of cool dialysate temperature dialysis in patients with frequent episodes of intradialytic hypotension [42, 43]. These guidelines also suggested that dialysate temperature below 35 °C should not be used. Increasing the time per session or by adding a fourth treatment per week can also be offered to patients with intradialytic hypotension. The pharmacologic option is HD patients with intradialytic hypotension include selective alpha-1 adrenergic agonist, midodrine. The optimal dose was not established, 2.5–5 mg 15–30 minutes prior to dialysis is usually given in the clinical practice [44]. An option for patients who have chronic, debilitating intradialytic hypotension could be switched to peritoneal dialysis, hemodiafiltration, or nocturnal dialysis, if available. Patients with intradialytic hypotension have increased morbidity and mortality [45]; in addition, hemodialysis with the episodes of hypotension is generally suboptimal due to earlier termination of the session, necessity of fluid replacement, problems with achieving target weight, etc. Fistula thrombosis is also more frequent in patients with hypotension. As intradialytic hypotension is a serious complication, it should be diagnosed and managed accordingly.

Renal Failure and Postprandial Hypotension

Postprandial blood pressure drop with larger meals with lot of simple carbohydrates is seen with meals with hemodialysis [46–48]. Intradialytic food intake may worsen the BP drop and may exacerbate the hemodialysis-related symptoms likes cramping, headaches, and nausea. Lack of caffeinated items such as coffee increases the risk of postprandial hypotension [49]. Some clinicians argue that food intake during dialysis may offer a supervised and effective therapy for protein energy wasting in renal failure subjects. Randomized controlled trials that balance the risks and benefits of eating are lacking [50].

Chronic Kidney Disease and Post-exercise Hypotension

In the laboratory settings, it was found in CKD subjects acute aerobic exercise leads to reduction in blood pressure for at least 60 minutes [51]. In predialysis patients, post-exercise hypotension is not seen with moderate intensity continuous aerobic training [52]. A small study in stages 2 and 3 of CKD showed hemodynamic and neural response benefit with aerobic exercise [53].

Chronic Kidney Disease and Nocturnal Hypotension

Hypotension episodes appear as a relatively common but underrecognized problem. As CKD is associated with abnormal pattern of BP changes in ABPM with extreme dippers or nondippers, it may contribute to worse cardiovascular outcomes [54, 55].

Conclusions

However, concerns about causing OH or its CVD consequences should not deter a lower BP goal among adults with chronic kidney disease attributed to hypertension as was shown recently [56]. Intradialytic hypotension should be evaluated promptly and managed timely as it is also associated with increased all-cause and cardiovascular mortality.

References

1. Sjostrand T. Volume and distribution of blood and their significance in regulating the circulation. Physiol Rev. 1953;33(2):202–28.
2. Shibao C, Lipsitz LA, Biaggioni I. Evaluation and treatment of orthostatic hypotension. J Am Soc Hypertens. 2013;7(4):317–24.
3. Briasoulis A, Silver A, Yano Y, Bakris GL. Orthostatic hypotension associated with baroreceptor dysfunction: treatment approaches. J Clin Hypertens (Greenwich). 2014;16(2): 141–8.
4. Freeman R, Wieling W, Axelrod FB, Benditt DG, Benarroch E, Biaggioni I, et al. Consensus statement on the definition of orthostatic hypotension, neurally mediated syncope and the postural tachycardia syndrome. Clin Auton Res. 2011;21(2):69–72.
5. Wożakowska-Kapłon B, Salwa P, Siebert J. New European guidelines on management of hypertension- do the change the clinical practice? Folia Cardiol. 2014;9:33–53.
6. Brignole M, Alboni P, Benditt DG, et al. The Task Force on Syncope, European Society of Cardiology. Guidelines on management (diagnosis and treatment) of syncope update 2004. Europace. 2004;6:467–537.
7. Banach M. Update on hypotension. Med Rodz. 2004;6:246–50.
8. Grześkowiak A, Rojek A, Szyndler A, et al. Pervalence of hypotension on hypertsive treatment. Nadciśn Tętn. 2005;9:452.
9. Poon IO, Braun U. High prevalence of orthostatic hypotension and its correlation potentially causative medications among elderly veterans. J Clin Pharm Ther. 2005;30:173–8.
10. Kario K. Orthostatic hypertension-a new haemodynamic cardiovascular risk factor. Nat Rev Nephrol. 2013;9(12):726–38.

11. Kurtal H, Schwenger V, Azzaro M, Abdollahnia N, Steinhagen-Thiessen E, Nieczaj R, Schulz RJ. Clinical value of automatic reporting of estimated glomerular filtration rate in geriatrics. Gerontology. 2009;55(3):288–95.

12. Malyszko J, Bachorzewska-Gajewska H, Malyszko JS, Dobrzycki S. Prevalence ofchronic kidney disease in elderly patients with normal serum creatinine levelsundergoing percutaneous coronary interventions. Gerontology. 2010;56(1):51–4.

13. Townsend RR, Chang TI, Cohen DL, Cushman WC, Evans GW, Glasser SP, Haley WE, Olney C, Oparil S, Del Pinto R, Pisoni R, Taylor AA, Umanath K, Wright JT Jr, Yeboah J, SPRINT Study Research Group. Orthostatic changes in systolic bloodpressure among SPRINT participants at baseline. J Am Soc Hypertens. 2016;10(11):847–56.

14. Franceschini N, Rose KM, Astor BC, Couper D, Vupputuri S. Orthostatichypotension and incident chronic kidney disease: the atherosclerosis risk incommunities study. Hypertension. 2010;56(6):1054–9.

15. Pacher P, Kecskemeti V. Cardiovascular side effects of new antidepressants and antipsychotics: new drugs, old concerns? Curr Pharm Des. 2004;10(20):2463–75.

16. Hugghins SY, Champion HC, Cheng G, Kadowitz PJ, Jeter JR Jr. Vasorelaxant responses to endomorphins, nociceptin, albuterol, and adrenomedullin in isolated rat aorta. Life Sci. 2000;67(4):471–6.

17. Barke KE, Hough LB. Opiates, mast cells and histamine release. Life Sci. 1993;53(18):1391–9.

18. Williams B, Mancia G, Spiering W, AgabitiRosei E, Azizi M, Burnier M, Clement DL, Coca A, de Simone G, Dominiczak A, Kahan T, Mahfoud F, Redon J, Ruilope L, Zanchetti A, Kerins M, Kjeldsen SE, Kreutz R, Laurent S, Lip GYH, McManus R, Narkiewicz K, Ruschitzka F, Schmieder RE, Shlyakhto E, Tsioufis C, Aboyans V, Desormais I, Authors/Task Force Members. 2018 ESC/ESH Guidelines for the management of arterial hypertension: the task force for the management ofarterial hypertension of the European Society of Cardiology and the European Society of Hypertension: the task force for the management of arterialhypertension of the European Society of Cardiology and the European society ofHypertension. J Hypertens. 2018;36(10):1953–2041.

19. Lewis JB. Blood pressure control in chronic kidney disease: is less really more? J Am Soc Nephrol. 2010;21:1086–92.

20. Hajjar I. Postural blood pressure changes and orthostatic hypotension in the elderly patient: impact of antihypertensive medications. Drugs Aging. 2005;22:55–68.

21. Tykocki T, Guzek K, Nauman P. Orthostatic hypotension and hypertension in supine in autonomic disorders. Pathophysiology, diagnosis and treatment. Kard Pol. 2010;68:1057–63.

22. Kooman J, Basci A, Pizzarelli F, et al. EBPG guideline on haemodynamic instability. Nephrol Dial Transplant. 2007;22(Suppl 2):ii22–44.

23. Sands JJ, Usvyat LA, Sullivan T, et al. Intradialytic hypotension: frequency, sources of variation and correlation with clinical outcome. Hemodial Int. 2014;18:415–22.

24. Reilly RF. Attending rounds: a patient with intradialytic hypotension. Clin J Am Soc Nephrol. 2014;9:798–803.

25. Santos SF, Peixoto AJ, Perazella MA. How should we manage adverse intradialytic blood pressure changes? Adv Chronic Kidney Dis. 2012;19:158–65.

26. van der Sande FM, Kooman JP, Leunissen KM. Intradialytic hypotension--new concepts on an old problem. Nephrol Dial Transplant. 2000;15:1746.

27. Flythe JE, Kunaparaju S, Dinesh K, et al. Factors associated with intradialytic systolic blood pressure variability. Am J Kidney Dis. 2012;59:409.

28. Henderson LW. Symptomatic hypotension during hemodialysis. Kidney Int. 1980;17:571–6.

29. Sinha AD, Agarwal R. Can chronic volume overload be recognized and prevented in hemodialysis patients? The pitfalls of the clinical examination in assessing volume status. Semin Dial. 2009;22:480–2.

30. Kouw PM, Kooman JP, Cheriex EC, et al. Assessment of postdialysis dry weight: a comparison of techniques. J Am Soc Nephrol. 1993;4:98.

31. Bégin V, Déziel C, Madore F. Biofeedback regulation of ultrafiltration and dialysate conductivity for the prevention of hypotension during hemodialysis. ASAIO J. 2002;48:312.
32. Brennan JM, Ronan A, Goonewardena S, et al. Handcarried ultrasound measurement of the inferior vena cava for assessment of intravascular volume status in the outpatient hemodialysis clinic. Clin J Am Soc Nephrol. 2006;1:749.
33. Mc Causland FR, Waikar SS. Association of predialysis calculated plasma osmolarity with intradialytic blood pressure decline. Am J Kidney Dis. 2015;66:499.
34. Ewing DJ, Winney R. Autonomic function in patients with chronic renal failure on intermittent haemodialysis. Nephron. 1975;15:424.
35. Daul AE, Wang XL, Michel MC, Brodde OE. Arterial hypotension in chronic hemodialyzed patients. Kidney Int. 1987;32:728.
36. Converse RL Jr, Jacobsen TN, Jost CM, et al. Paradoxical withdrawal of reflex vasoconstriction as a cause of hemodialysis-induced hypotension. J Clin Invest. 1992;90:1657.
37. Barnas MG, Boer WH, Koomans HA. Hemodynamic patterns and spectral analysis of heart rate variability during dialysis hypotension. J Am Soc Nephrol. 1999;10:2577.
38. Nette RW, van den Dorpel MA, Krepel HP, et al. Hypotension during hemodialysis results from an impairment of arteriolar tone and left ventricular function. Clin Nephrol. 2005;63:276.
39. Poldermans D, Man in't Veld AJ, Rambaldi R, et al. Cardiac evaluation in hypotension-prone and hypotension-resistant hemodialysis patients. Kidney Int. 1999;56:1905.
40. Kolb J, Kitzler TM, Tauber T, et al. Proto-dialytic cardiac function relates to intra-dialytic morbid events. Nephrol Dial Transplant. 2011;26:1645.
41. Jindal K, Chan CT, Deziel C, et al. Hemodialysis clinical practice guidelines for the Canadian Society of Nephrology. J Am Soc Nephrol. 2006;17:S1.
42. K/DOQI Workgroup. K/DOQI clinical practice guidelines for cardiovascular disease in dialysis patients. Am J Kidney Dis. 2005;45:S1.
43. Tattersall J, Martin-Malo A, Pedrini L, et al. EBPG guideline on dialysis strategies. Nephrol Dial Transplant. 2007;22(Suppl 2):ii5.
44. Cruz DN, Mahnensmith RL, Perazella MA. Intradialytic hypotension: is midodrine beneficial in symptomatic hemodialysis patients. Am J Kidney Dis. 1997;30:772–9.
45. Flythe JE, Inrig JK, Shafi T, Chang TI, Cape K, Dinesh K, Kunaparaju S, Brunelli SM. Association of intradialytic blood pressure variability with increased all-cause and cardiovascular mortality in patients treated with long-term hemodialysis. Am J Kidney Dis. 2013;61:966–74.
46. Borzou SR, Mahdipour F, Oshvandi K, Salavati M, Alimohammadi N. Effect of mealtime during hemodialysis on patients' complications. J Caring Sci. 2016;5:277–86.
47. Sherman RA, Torres F, Cody RP. Postprandial blood pressure changes during hemodialysis. Am J Kidney Dis. 1988;12:37–9.
48. Sivalingam M, Banerjee A, Nevett G, Farrington K. Haemodynamic effects of food intake during haemodialysis. Blood Purif. 2008;26:157–62.
49. Barakat MM, Nawab ZM, Yu AW, Lau AH, Ing TS, Daugirdas JT. Hemodynamic effects of intradialytic food ingestion and the effects of caffeine. J Am Soc Nephrol. 1993;3:1813–8.
50. Agarwal R, Georgianos P. Feeding during dialysis- risks and uncertainties. Nephrol Dial Transplant. 2018;33:917–22.
51. Headley SAJ, Germain MJ, Milch CM, Bichholz MP, Coughlin MA, Pescatello LS. Immediate blood pressure lowering effects of aerobic exercise among patients with chronic kidney disease. Nephrology (Carlton). 2008;13:601–6.
52. Headley S, Germain M, Wood R, Joubert J, Milch C, Evans E, Cornelius A, Brewer B, Taylor B, Pescatello LS. Blood pressure response to acute and chronic exercise in chronic kidney disease. Nephrology (Carlton). 2017;22:72–8.
53. April DC, Oneda B, Gusmao JL, Costa LA, Forjaz CL, Mion D Jr, Tinucci T. Post-exercise hypotension is mediated by a decrease in sympathetic nerve activity in stages 2-3 CKD. Am J Nephrol. 2016;43:206–12.

54. Fagard RH, Celis H, Thijs L, et al. Daytime and nighttime blood pres- sure as predictors of death and cause-specific cardiovascular events in hypertension. Hypertension. 2008;51:55–61.
55. Yano Y, Kario K. Nocturnal blood pressure and cardiovascular disease: a review of recent advances. Hypertens Res. 2012;35:695–701.
56. Juraschek SP, Appel LJ, Miller ER 3rd, Mukamal KJ, Lipsitz LA. Hypertension treatment effects on orthostatic hypotension and its relationship with cardiovascular disease. Hypertension. 2018;72(4):986–93.

Stroke and Hypotensive Syndromes

14

Mariusz Stasiolek

Introduction

Due to the impending changes in demographic structure, geriatric syndromes (dementia, depression, falls, urinary incontinence, functional decline, decreased hearing, and vision) represent growing medical and socioeconomical problem in modern societies. The etiopathology of particular geriatric syndromes remains to be fully elucidated. However, the growing body of evidence indicates vascular changes as an important common causative factor. Vascular aging and dysfunction together with large and small vessel disease as well as cardiac pathology may lead to recurrent focal and global brain ischemic events. These in turn may present clinically as symptomatic stroke episodes or have an asymptomatic course of "silent infarction." Importantly, the chronic accumulation of ischemic brain damage and associated neurodegenerative processes play a crucial role in the pathogenesis of white matter disease or leukoaraiosis, which severity in turn seems to be correlated with the burden of geriatric syndromes [3]. Taking into consideration brain physiology, recurrent hypotension may potentially aggravate the detrimental effects of vascular impairment in elderly in the context of progressively accumulated cerebral ischemic lesions and neurodegeneration. It may also increase the risk of acute ischemic stroke in the mechanisms described in the following sections.

Stroke Definitions

The pathophysiology of stroke is complex and heterogeneous and therefore the definition of "stroke" has to be clearly outlined at the beginning of this chapter. The World Health Organization (WHO) definition from 1970 describes stroke as "rapidly developing clinical signs of focal (or global) disturbance of cerebral function,

M. Stasiolek (✉)
Department of Neurology, Medical University of Lodz, Lodz, Poland

© Springer Nature Switzerland AG 2020   139
K. Alagiakrishnan, M. Banach (eds.), *Hypotensive Syndromes in Geriatric Patients*, https://doi.org/10.1007/978-3-030-30332-7_14

lasting more than 24 hours or leading to death, with no apparent cause other than that of vascular origin" [2]. However, thanks to the significantly better understanding of stroke pathology as well as substantial development of medical technology allowing for increasingly more effective central nervous system (CNS) tissue and vasculature imaging, the definition of stroke has been evolving. The group of experts from American Heart Association and American Stroke Association (AHA and ASA) issued in 2013 new set of definitions based on the analysis of available clinical, neuroimaging, and pathophysiological data. In this consensus document, the term "stroke" is advised to be understood broadly in reference to ischemic stroke, stroke caused by intracerebral hemorrhage, stroke caused by subarachnoid hemorrhage, stroke caused by cerebral venous thrombosis, or stroke not otherwise specified when an episode of acute neurological dysfunction is presumed to be caused by ischemia or hemorrhage (but without sufficient evidence) and persists ≥24 hours or until death. Ischemic stroke is defined as an episode of neurological dysfunction caused by focal cerebral, spinal, or retinal infarction. Next to the *exclusion of global ischemia* from the stroke spectrum, significant novelty is brought in this area by the detailed definition of CNS infarction. According to the AHA/ASA definition, CNS infarction is brain, spinal cord, or retinal cell death attributable to ischemia, based on (1) pathological, imaging, or other objective evidence of cerebral, spinal cord, or retinal focal ischemic injury in a defined vascular distribution or (2) clinical evidence of cerebral, spinal cord, or retinal focal ischemic injury based on symptoms persisting ≥24 hours or until death, and other etiologies excluded. The clearly specified *acknowledgment of "tissue/imaging" factor* allowed for the inclusion of silent CNS infarction, described as imaging or neuropathological evidence of CNS infarction, without a history of acute neurological dysfunction attributable to the lesion among stroke modalities [74].

Also, the definition of transient ischemic attack (TIA) has been modified due to similar considerations as in the case of stroke [22]. In consequence, the current AHA/ASA definition recognizes the importance of tissue damage criterion and describes TIA as a transient episode of neurological dysfunction caused by focal brain, spinal cord, or retinal ischemia, without acute infarction. The duration of TIA symptoms, which is very important, is not specified in this definition [22].

The new AHA/ASA definitions evoke, however, significant controversy in regard to implementation in everyday clinical practice. The limited sensitivity and specificity of modern neuroimaging techniques are pointed at together with the substantial risk of overtreatment of "silent strokes" and undertreatment of cases with negative imaging profile [1].

Stroke Mechanisms and Risk Factors

Stroke is a major cause of disability and the second leading preventable death cause worldwide [89]. According to "AHA 2016 statistical update," overall stroke prevalence was 2.6% in US population > 20 years of age. Apart from age, the main nonmodifiable risk factor of stroke, the prevalence and incidence depended on race, level of education, and geographical differences [56]. High blood pressure, diabetes mellitus, disorders of heart rhythm, high blood level of cholesterol and other lipids, smoking/tobacco use, physical inactivity, nutritional factors, family history and genetics, chronic kidney disease, and psychosocial factors are listed among the main risk factors of stroke [56]. Importantly, the results provided by the INTERSTROKE study, performed in 32 low- to high-income countries, indicate that the same factors contribute to the risk of stroke all over the world [59]. Hypertension, physical inactivity, apolipoprotein (Apo)B/ApoA1 ratio, diet, waist-to-hip ratio, psychosocial factors, current smoking, cardiac causes, alcohol consumption, and diabetes mellitus were associated with all stroke and accounted for more than 90% of the population attributable risks. Among them, previous history of hypertension was the most important of the modifiable risk factors [41].

The TIA criteria used in particular studies may strongly influence the epidemiological data. However, consistent observations indicate that the incidence of TIA increases with age regardless of race and gender and reaches in some cohorts >85 years of age values exceeding 10 cases per 1000 per year, which is of great importance considering the association of TIA with subsequent stroke. Increased short- and long-term risk of stroke after TIA was demonstrated in multiple studies. Over 10% of patients will experience stroke in 90 days after TIA with the greatest short-term risk within the first 2 days. The risk of subsequent stroke can be stratified with particular scales, e.g., ABCD2 score, including such variables as age > 60 years, blood pressure > 140/90 mmHg, clinical symptoms, duration, and diabetes. Additionally, changes in brain imaging as well as intracranial or extracranial stenosis were associated with an increased stroke risk in TIA patients [22].

Regardless of the accomplished and impending changes in the definition of stroke, the main causes of stroke are cerebral ischemia, intracerebral hemorrhage, and subarachnoid hemorrhage, responsible for ca. 87%, 10%, and 3%, respectively, of stroke cases in the United States [56]. Based on the pathophysiological mechanisms, cerebral ischemia may be divided into several main subtypes: (1) thrombotic stroke (with subtypes typical for large or small vessel occlusion), (2) embolic stroke, (3) watershed or border zone stroke, and (4) stroke secondary to venous thrombosis [20]. Importantly, in clinical settings, ca. one third of TIA and acute ischemic stroke cases remain of undetermined cause referred to as cryptogenic stroke [46]. Severely diminished blood supply to the brain regions is the common denominator of all the ischemic stroke subtypes. Although theoretically possible, CNS hypoperfusion due to the systemic hypotension as cause of stroke continues to evoke some controversy. This mechanism is postulated mainly in the pathophysiology of border zone stroke.

The term watershed or border zone stroke applies to ischemic lesions in an area localized between distal fields of two nonanastomosing arterial systems. The supratentorial watershed regions may be divided into cortical (external) and subcortical (internal) border zone. According to clinical, anatomopathological, and experimental data, recurrent episodes of severe systemic hypotension may result in hemodynamic failure in the watershed areas especially localized distal to severe arterial stenosis or occlusion. Due to the anatomical conditions, the internal border zone is regarded more vulnerable to hemodynamic impairment. Additionally, the risk of such ischemic lesions in the territory of middle cerebral artery grows in the situation of malfunctional circle of Willis [50, 55]. Although the hemodynamic theory seems to be sufficiently documented, microembolic mechanism of water-shed infarcts has been also postulated particularly in cortical border zone [7, 21]. It is however plausible that in some patients, both mechanisms could coexist in the pathology of border zone infarction. Cardiac disease or severe internal carotid artery stenosis is often associated with both microembolism and profound hemo-dynamic impairment. In consequence, watershed areas characterized by least per-fusion pressure may be particularly susceptible to the impaired emboli clearance and its detrimental effects [50, 55].

The issue of the possible influence of systemic hypotension on the risk of stroke was examined in the last years particularly in the context of intensive blood pressure lowering therapies. Although large clinical trials did not confirm unequivocally the association, some of the observational studies indicate that the risk of stroke increased in patients with diastolic hypotension [10, 73].

Blood Pressure and Acute Stroke

From the pathophysiological point of view, it is important to understand that the cerebral blood flow (CBF) is determined by the ratio of arterial pressure and vas-culature resistance. CBF has to be in a stable manner adjusted to the high level of brain metabolism and the homeostasis is maintained thanks to the autoregulation mechanisms specific for cerebral vasculature. The level of resistance is modified according to changes in perfusion pressure as well as in response to chemical sig-nals associated with physiological local metabolic fluctuations or generated by pathological processes, e.g., ischemia. Autonomic innervation exerts much lower effects on cerebral vasculature than in other organs [68]. This characteristic bears special meaning in the situation of acute brain infarction. The reactive maximal dilatation of vasculature in the core ischemic areas and the failure to exert appro-priate vasoconstrictive response render CBF crucially dependent on mean arterial pressure [68]. Also in moderately hypoperfused area of ischemic penumbra, ade-quately high blood pressure seems to be vital for formation and maintenance of pressure gradients enabling collateral blood flow through the collateral circulation. However, very high values and/or sudden increase of systemic blood pressure may reduce CBF and contribute to blood-brain barrier damage, edema formation, and hemorrhagic transformation [44].

The current 2018 AHA/ASA guidelines provide a new recommendation in acute ischemic stroke stating that "Hypotension and hypovolemia should be corrected to maintain systemic perfusion levels necessary to support organ function." However, because of lack of conclusive data, the suggestions regarding the treatment of low blood pressure in patients with stroke are not specified in the publication [66]. Individualized attempt to patients with very high blood pressure values is sug-gested with emphasis laid on comorbid conditions and eligibility for recanalyzing therapy application [66]. Although, no sufficient data are available on the exact values of optimal blood pressure [66], U-shaped association between admission blood pressure and unfavorable outcome of acute ischemic stroke was suggested in retrospective and prospective studies [12, 84]. Importantly, in a recent prospective analysis of patients with first-ever ischemic stroke, not only very high blood pressure values but also mean admission blood pressure < 100 mmHg and discharge systolic blood pressure < 120 mmHg were associated with increased all-cause mortality [90]. Other clinical trials assessing the influence of blood pressure modulation in acute phase of ischemic stroke showed inconsistent and even conflicting results, which did not allow for conclusive assessment in meta-analyses performed till now [31, 32]. The lack of sufficient evidence in this area may be at least partially explained by the comorbidities influencing the outcome of blood pressure modification but also by complexity of brain infarction pathophysiology with different subtypes of stroke, volume of the core and penumbra in particular cases, and the conditions of the compensatory perfusion maintenance and availability of collateral vessels in the penumbra as well as the status of revascularization gained in acute phase of infarction [12, 47, 68]. In this model, very high blood pressure in the acute phase may suggest systemic reaction to poor collateralization, large vessel occlusion, and large infarction volume. Accordingly, spontaneous decrease in blood pressure values was shown to correlate with recanalization success, smaller infarction, and better outcome in acute ischemic stroke patients [12, 52]. In contrast, very low blood pressure associated mainly with systemic circulatory failure may result in insufficient collateral blood flow in hypoperfused brain tissue and poor prognosis [12]. The introduction of intravenous thrombolysis and recently also mechanical endovascular procedures to everyday clinical practice in stroke units [66] increased the complexity of blood pressure control in acute ischemic stroke. In the light of the above-mentioned observations, target blood pressure values should be adjusted to the recanalization status (pre- vs. postrecanalization procedure) in acute phase and to multiple clinical factors including reperfusion outcome and the risk of hemorrhagic conversion in further stages [12, 51, 87]. Available data indicate again that both high and low or dropping blood pressure values, e.g., in connection with general anesthesia during endovascular stroke treatment, may be associated with poor outcome [88]. However, still the amount of data is not satisfactory for definitive conclusions [12, 68, 78].

Contrary to cerebral ischemia, in the case of hemorrhagic stroke, there is a common trend among clinicians to lower high blood pressure in order to decrease the risk of hematoma expansion. However, randomized clinical trials investigating the effect of intensive vs. moderate blood pressure reduction in acute phase of hemorrhagic stroke did not show conclusive results. Based on that, AHA and European Stroke Organisation (ESO) issued guidelines stating that in spontaneous intracerebral hemorrhage, early lowering of systolic blood pressure to <140 mmHg is well tolerated and may improve functional outcome [34, 80]. Recently two independent meta-analyses of randomized controlled clinical trials were published – each encompassing data from more than 4000 patients with spontaneous intracerebral hemorrhage. The results showed no differences between aggressive and conservative blood pressure lowering in major outcome measures [33, 79].

However, significant decrease in hematoma growth was found in one of the sub-group analyses in younger patients (age $\leq$ 62 years) with smaller hematoma volume ($\leq$15 mL) treated within 6 hours [79]. In the other meta-analysis, lower rate of unfavorable outcomes was described in patients with no history of hypertension, or longer prehospital duration, or lower NIHSS score [33]. Importantly, the rate of renal adverse event in intensive treatment group was found significantly higher in this analysis [33].

Stroke and Orthostatic Hypotension

Orthostatic hypotension (OH) is a failure of cardiovascular reflexes to maintain blood pressure on standing from supine or sitting position. According to consensus guideline, OH is defined as a decrease in systolic blood pressure of at least 20 mmHg and/or diastolic blood pressure of at least 10 mmHg within 3 minutes of standing [18]. Typical symptoms of OH are mostly referable to cerebral hypoperfusion and include positional dizziness, presyncope or syncope, dimmed or blurred vision, weakness of the legs, headache, cognitive slowing, and tiredness. Because of the sudden drops of blood pressure, OH patients are also believed to be more prone to experience falls [28, 53]. However, in the great proportion of detected cases, OH may remain asymptomatic. Moreover, the cardiovascular response to orthostatic challenge may differ over time, and in some patients, OH can be transient in opposition to patients with confirmed persistent OH [11]. Although different in various populations, the prevalence of OH increases significantly with age and affects 10–30% of the elderly [49]. The elevated prevalence of OH in older persons can be explained by the gradual impairment of the blood pressure control system associated with increase in vascular stiffness and decrease of baroreflex sensitivity and beta-adrenoreceptor-mediated responses as well as with improper volume and nutritional status and the presence of associated conditions [11, 48]. Aging is associated with increased number of several comorbidities that influence significantly the prevalence of OH such as neurodegenerative disorders (e.g., Parkinson's disease, dementia with Lewy bodies, multisystem atrophy), diabetes, hypertension, congestive cardiac failure, prior myocardial infarction, carotid artery disease, various forms of autonomic neuropathy, and postacute illness [11, 16]. Of great importance is the fact that also the medications administered commonly in elderly patients may induce and/or exacerbate OH. It applies particularly to different types of antihypertensive drugs but also to alpha-adrenoreceptor antagonists (as therapy of benign prostatic hyperplasia), tricyclic antidepressants, vasodilatators, sympatholytics, and antiparkinsonian agents (L-DOPA, dopamine receptor agonists) [11, 54]. Additive effects of different classes of potentially causative medications in OH have been suggested [65]. Noteworthy, current smoking was indicated as a factor linked to higher OH prevalence [26].

Over the last 20 years, multiple prospective studies performed on European, North American, and Asiatic populations analyzed the association between OH and the risk of cardiovascular disease, cognitive decline, falls, and all-cause mortality

[6]. The studies performed on various populations with different methodology gave partially inconsistent results. However, a significant association of OH with all-cause mortality and cardiovascular events was shown in the majority of the studies assessing these parameters [6]. Among various cardiovascular conditions, stroke belongs to the most frequently investigated in association with OH. Again, the results of particular prospective epidemiological studies performed on different populations with different follow-up time are not consistent [4, 13, 23, 26, 27, 72, 86]. Importantly, in some of the analyses, the effect of OH on the risk of stroke was completely abolished after adjustment to confounders such as age, gender, systolic blood pressure, diabetes mellitus, and smoking – regarded as independent cardiovascular risk factors [13, 26]. In other studies, age-dependent influence of OH on the risk of future stroke was observed [23, 86]. The recent meta-analysis summarized current evidence regarding the association between OH and cardiovascular disease including coronary heart disease and stroke [91]. The analysis encompassed 7 cohort studies with over 64,000 participants who were free of coronary heart disease and stroke at baseline, with mean follow-up time over 15 years. The results showed significant effect of OH on the risk of investigated cardiovascular conditions. The presence of OH at baseline increased the risk of stroke both in middle-aged (< 65 years) and older participants. Most importantly, possible confounding factors such as age, gender, mean BMI, hypertension, and diabetes did not seem to affect the prospective association between OH and incidental stroke. Additionally, association between OH and ischemic stroke seemed to be stronger than in the case of all stroke events [91]. These results stay in line with the pathophysiology of different types of stroke and underline the need of further studies directed on specific cerebrovascular pathology.

Lately, results of about 25–26 years of follow-up of the Atherosclerosis Risk in Communities (ARIC) cohort were published [23, 37, 67]. One of the analyses included data obtained from ca. 12,000 participants and revealed that patients with OH at baseline had higher risk of dementia and ischemic stroke [67]. The other analysis performed on the population of ca. 9000 ARIC participants concentrated on various cardiovascular conditions and presented strong association of OH with future risk of stroke, myocardial infarction, congestive heart failure, and fatal coronary heart disease as well as carotid intimal thickness and carotid plaque. The association was independent of wide spectrum of established cardiovascular risk factors [37].

Much less is known about the influence of cerebral ischemia on hypotension and in particular OH. However, there are reports indicating that chronic stroke may be associated with complex autonomic and vascular dysfunction attenuating cardiovascular response to standing and affecting cerebral blood flow velocity regulation [58, 70].

These data represent substantial evidence supporting OH as an important, and very common among elderly persons, risk factor of cerebrovascular complications. Moreover, it can be assumed that at least in some cases, OH indicates coexistence of early subclinical cardiovascular disease in the patient [37] and consequently should be considered as reason for further thorough health assessment. However, the exact interrelation between OH and other cardiovascular risk factors has yet to be sufficiently elucidated in large epidemiological studies. The strong influence of established cardiovascular risk factors on OH prevalence makes it still possible that OH acts rather as a marker of cardiovascular burden and not as a risk factor by itself. Discerning of these two possibilities would have a substantial impact on therapeutic approach in the elderly, e.g., in regard to aggressive hypertension treatment.

Stroke and Postprandial Hypotension

Postprandial hypotension (PPH) is defined mostly as a fall of ≥20 mmHg in systolic blood pressure occurring within 2 hours of a meal and persisting for at least 30 minutes [36]. However, the definition varies across scientific sources mainly in regard to the scheme of blood pressure measurement [62]. Commonly described clinical manifestations of PPH are attributed to cerebral hypoperfusion and include dizzines, nausea, light-headedness, and visual disturbances [62]. The condition has been studied mostly in the elderly and reported in up to 40% of "healthy" older persons [83]. The prevalence tends to correlate with frailty and increases in disorders affecting the function of autonomic nervous system such as diabetes and neurodegenerative conditions, e.g., Parkinson's disease. The recent meta-analysis of 11 case-controlled studies showed that there is a significantly increased likelihood of PPH in patients suffering from diabetes, Parkinson's disease, multisystem atrophy, and Alzheimer's disease [62]. On the other hand, PPH is considered as an independent risk factor for falls, coronary events, and all-cause mortality [8, 29, 57]. Importantly, PPH was also associated with an increased risk of the asymptomatic cerebrovascular damage (lacunar infarction and leukoaraiosis) [42, 81] and new symptomatic stroke incidents in older persons [8]. The mechanisms underlying the possible effect of PPH on cerebral ischemia have not been sufficiently investigated. It is however plausible that sudden drop in systemic blood pressure may be accompanied by insufficient or even paradoxical reaction of brain vasculature [43]. This in turn could be explained by both vascular aging and by dysfunctional autonomic regulation secondary to accumulated brain pathology in older patients.

Taking in consideration the very high prevalence of PPH in the elderly and its coexistence with multiple cardiovascular risk factors, further studies are definitely needed in order to properly evaluate the most probably bidirectional association of PPH and cerebrovascular pathology. In this context also the possible impact of PPH on poststroke therapy and physical rehabilitation of older patients needs to be carefully investigated [25].

Stroke and Nocturnal Hypotension

The exact prognostic significance of circadian blood pressure changes in the risk profile of cardiovascular diseases remains to be fully elucidated. Inconsistent results were reported in this area by several prospective epidemiologic studies evaluating the association of various measures of daytime and nighttime blood pressure with the risk of multiple conditions including myocardial infarction, coronary heart disease, congestive heart failure, peripheral arterial disease, sudden death as well as stroke and TIA [9, 19, 24, 35, 63, 64, 85]. Elevated nocturnal blood pressure or the lack of nocturnal blood pressure dipping and so-called reverse-dipping pattern were shown in some of the analyses as independent predictors of cardiovascular disease. However, the contrary pattern of nocturnal blood pressure change – the so-called extreme-dipper pattern – was also identified as a risk factor for cerebrovascular disease by some of the authors [17, 75]. Noteworthy, J-shaped relation was described between nocturnal blood pressure dipping status and both silent cerebral ischemia [38] and symptomatic stroke in older hypertensive patients [39]. Interestingly, the extreme-dipper group in this study presented also tendency to higher percentages of ischemic strokes that occurred during sleep [39]. Recently, the results of The Ambulatory Blood Pressure Collaboration in Patients With Hypertension Meta-Analysis were published [75]. The meta-analysis encompassed 10 cohorts with over 17,000 hypertensive patients. The nocturnal blood pressure changes were correlated with fatal and nonfatal cardiovascular events including coronary heart disease events and stroke, cardiovascular mortality, and all-cause mortality. The systolic night-to-day ratio and reverse dipping predicted all end points, while in the case of extreme dippers, the results depended on the treatment status of hypertension. Interestingly, among treated patients, extreme dipping carried no increased risk, whereas among untreated cohorts, it was associated with an elevation of the risk for total cardiovascular events similar to reverse dippers [75].

Although the mechanisms underlying the influence of nocturnal hypotension on the development of cerebrovascular pathology are not sufficiently known, it is assumed that extreme dippers tend to have predominant systolic hypertension and increased blood pressure variability. Additionally, nocturnal hypotension may be associated with increased arterial stiffness, reduced circulating blood volume, and decreased cerebral perfusion, especially in older persons [40, 69]. The other possible mechanism is an excessive morning blood pressure surge due to alpha-adrenergic hyperactivity [40].

The above-mentioned observations underscore the importance of assessment of circadian blood pressure changes in planning of therapy in patients with cardiovascular disease. Few studies performed in groups of stroke survivors provide additional information in this regard. In acute stroke settings, nocturnal blood pressure dipping pattern was not associated with functional outcome at 3 months in ca. 300 patients treated with intravenous thrombolysis [76]. Similarly in an earlier analysis, performed in the first 48 hours post acute stroke, there was no clear influence of dipping pattern on the rate of death or dependency at 3 months [60]. In another study, reverse dipper and high nighttime heart rate detected in the first 2 weeks post acute stroke were associated with total mortality during long-term follow-up, while extreme dipping did not show such association [61]. However, nocturnal hypotension incidents were detected in the majority of a group of 63 poststroke patients independent of age, sex, vascular risk factors, or antihypertensive treatment administered [15]. Interestingly, one of the studies demonstrated that the blunting of normal diurnal variation in blood pressure was less pronounced in lacunar than in nonlacunar ischemic strokes [14], what may add to the complexity of the blood pressure control in patients with cerebral ischemia.

Stroke and Other Hypotensive Syndromes

The knowledge about the interrelation between stroke and other hypotensive syndromes is rather limited.

Vasovagal syncope is a neurally mediated reflex syncope caused by systemic arterial hypotension resulting from improper reflex reaction characterized by a lack of sympathetic vasoconstriction and/or a vagally mediated bradycardia. The most common precipitants include orthostatic stress (prolonged standing) but also emotional distress, pain, and gastrointestinal stimulation. Typical for reflex syncope are preceding vegetative symptoms (pallor, nausea, sweating, pupillary dilation) which can be less pronounced in the elderly [5, 71, 82]. In atypical cases of vasovagal syncope, prodromal symptoms can be absent or be constricted to blurred vision, fatigue, and pallor. Sometimes paresthesiae are reported – especially by women. During syncopal phase, clonic jerks and incontinence can be present. Retrograde amnesia can complicate the postictal phase particularly in older persons [5, 77, 82]. Another form of reflex syncope – carotid sinus syncope – occurs mainly in older persons and is regarded as one of the main causes of sudden falls. Carotid sinus syncope is often evoked by turning movements of the head or the neck compression [5, 82].

In the cases of transient loss of consciousness accompanied by additional neurologic symptoms and signs, it is important to differentiate with vertebrobasilar TIA and steal syndromes or epileptic seizures [71, 82]. It is of note that carotid sinus syndrome may be potentially associated with carotid artery pathology [30] and thus indirectly indicate an increased risk of cerebrovascular complications by hypotonic incidents.

There is not enough information in the literature about *post-exercise hypotension* in order to conclude about the interrelation with stroke. The available data indicate, however, that the physical exercise in poststroke patients causes reductions in diastolic blood pressure and nighttime systolic blood pressure, which can be helpful in the efficient nonpharmacological hypertension management [45].

Conclusions

Although the evidence regarding the association between stroke and hypotensive syndromes has been growing in the last decades, it is still not complete or even fragmentary in multiple areas. The understanding of the role of particular hypotensive syndromes in the risk profile of cerebrovascular events is complicated by the coexistence of various established cardiovascular risk factors, typical in the elderly. Also, the diverse pathophysiology of different types of stroke contributes to the complexity of this issue. However, regardless of the exact meaning as a risk factor of stroke or a cardiovascular burden marker, hypotensive syndromes have to be considered as important modulators of health and quality of life in the elderly. Consequently, hypotensive syndromes should be actively looked for, detected early, and taken into consideration in therapy planning and control in elderly patients.

References

1. Abbott AL, Silvestrini M, Topakian R, Golledge J, Brunser AM, de Borst GJ, Harbaugh RE, Doubal FN, Rundek T, Thapar A, Davies AH, Kam A, Wardlaw JM. Optimizing the definitions of stroke, transient ischemic attack, and infarction for research and application in clinical practice. Front Neurol. 2017;8:537. https://doi.org/10.3389/fneur.2017.00537. eCollection 2017.
2. Aho K, Harmsen P, Hatano S, Marquardsen J, Smirnov VE, Strasser T. Cerebrovascular disease in the community: results of a WHO collaborative study. Bull World Health Organ. 1980;58(1):113–30.
3. Alagiakrishnan K, Hsueh J, Zhang E, Khan K, Senthilselvan A. White matter disease severity of the brain and its association with geriatric syndromes. Postgrad Med. 2013;125(6):17–23. https://doi.org/10.3810/pgm.2013.11.2708.
4. Alagiakrishnan K, Patel K, Desai RV, Ahmed MB, Fonarow GC, Forman DE, White M, Aban IB, Love TE, Aronow WS, Allman RM, Anker SD, Ahmed A. Orthostatic hypotension and incident heart failure in community-dwelling older adults. J Gerontol A Biol Sci Med Sci. 2014;69(2):223–30. https://doi.org/10.1093/gerona/glt086.
5. Alboni P. The different clinical presentations of vasovagal syncope. Heart. 2015;101(9):674–8. https://doi.org/10.1136/heartjnl-2014-307096.
6. Angelousi A, Girerd N, Benetos A, Frimat L, Gautier S, Weryha G, Boivin JM. Association between orthostatic hypotension and cardiovascular risk, cerebrovascular risk, cognitive decline and falls as well as overall mortality: a systematic review and meta-analysis. J Hypertens. 2014;32(8):1562–71. https://doi.org/10.1097/HJH.0000000000000235.
7. Arakawa S, Minematsu K, Hirano T, Tanaka Y, Hasegawa Y, Hayashida K, Yamaguchi T. Topographic distribution of misery perfusion in relation to internal and superficial borderzones. AJNR Am J Neuroradiol. 2003;24(3):427–35.
8. Aronow WS, Ahn C. Association of postprandial hypotension with incidence of falls, syncope, coronary events, stroke, and total mortality at 29-month follow-up in 499 older nursing home residents. J Am Geriatr Soc. 1997;45(9):1051–3.
9. Bastos JM, Bertoquini S, Polónia J. Prognostic value of subdivisions of nighttime blood pressure fall in hypertensives followed up for 8.2 years. Does nondipping classification need to be redefined? J Clin Hypertens (Greenwich). 2010;12(7):508–15. https://doi.org/10.1111/j.1751-7176.2010.00291.x.
10. Bavishi C, Bangalore S, Messerli FH. Outcomes of intensive blood pressure lowering in older hypertensive patients. J Am Coll Cardiol. 2017;69(5):486–93. https://doi.org/10.1016/j.jacc.2016.10.077.
11. Benvenuto LJ, Krakoff LR. Morbidity and mortality of orthostatic hypotension: implications for management of cardiovascular disease. Am J Hypertens. 2011;24(2):135–44. https://doi.org/10.1038/ajh.2010.146.
12. Bösel J. Blood pressure control for acute severe ischemic and hemorrhagic stroke. Curr Opin Crit Care. 2017;23(2):81–6. https://doi.org/10.1097/MCC.0000000000000394.
13. Casiglia E, Tikhonoff V, Caffi S, Boschetti G, Giordano N, Guidotti F, Segato F, Mazza A, Grasselli C, Saugo M, Rigoni G, Guglielmi F, Martini B, Palatini P. Orthostatic hypotension does not increase cardiovascular risk in the elderly at a population level. Am J Hypertens. 2014;27(1):81–8. https://doi.org/10.1093/ajh/hpt172.

14. Castilla-Guerra L, Espino-Montoro A, Fernández-Moreno MC, López-Chozas JM. Abnormal blood pressure circadian rhythm in acute ischaemic stroke: are lacunar strokes really different? Int J Stroke. 2009;4(4):257–61. https://doi.org/10.1111/j.1747-4949.2009.00314.x.

15. Castilla-Guerra L, Fernandez-Moreno MC. Antihypertensive treatment after ischemic stroke in elderly adults: beware of nocturnal hypotension episodes. J Am Geriatr Soc. 2015;63(10):2204–5. https://doi.org/10.1111/jgs.13686.

16. Chisholm P, Anpalahan M. Orthostatic hypotension: pathophysiology, assessment, treatment and the paradox of supine hypertension. Intern Med J. 2017;47(4):370–9. https://doi.org/10.1111/imj.13171.

17. Coca A, Camafort M, Doménech M, Sierra C. Ambulatory blood pressure in stroke and cognitive dysfunction. Curr Hypertens Rep. 2013;15(3):150–9. https://doi.org/10.1007/s11906-013-0346-3.

18. Consensus statement on the definition of orthostatic hypotension, pure autonomic failure, and multiple system atrophy. The Consensus Committee of the American Autonomic Society and the American Academy of Neurology. Neurology. 1996;46(5):1470.

19. de la Sierra A, Banegas JR, Segura J, Gorostidi M, Ruilope LM, CARDIORISC Event Investigators. Ambulatory blood pressure monitoring and development of cardiovascular events in high-risk patients included in the Spanish ABPM registry: the CARDIORISC Event study. J Hypertens. 2012;30(4):713–9. https://doi.org/10.1097/HJH.0b013e328350bb40.

20. Deb P, Sharma S, Hassan KM. Pathophysiologic mechanisms of acute ischemic stroke: an overview with emphasis on therapeutic significance beyond thrombolysis. Pathophysiology. 2010;17(3):197–218. https://doi.org/10.1016/j.pathophys.2009.12.001.

21. Derdeyn CP, Khosla A, Videen TO, Fritsch SM, Carpenter DL, Grubb RL Jr, Powers WJ. Severe hemodynamic impairment and border zone--region infarction. Radiology. 2001;220(1):195–201.

22. Easton JD, Saver JL, Albers GW, Alberts MJ, Chaturvedi S, Feldmann E, Hatsukami TS, Higashida RT, Johnston SC, Kidwell CS, Lutsep HL, Miller E, Sacco RL, American Heart Association, American Stroke Association Stroke Council, Council on Cardiovascular Surgery and Anesthesia, Council on Cardiovascular Radiology and Intervention, Council on Cardiovascular Nursing, Interdisciplinary Council on Peripheral Vascular Disease. Definition and evaluation of transient ischemic attack: a scientific statement for healthcare professionals from the American Heart Association/American Stroke Association Stroke Council; Council on Cardiovascular Surgery and Anesthesia; Council on Cardiovascular Radiology and Intervention; Council on Cardiovascular Nursing; and the Interdisciplinary Council on Peripheral Vascular Disease. The American Academy of Neurology affirms the value of this statement as an educational tool for neurologists. Stroke. 2009;40(6):2276–93. https://doi.org/10.1161/STROKEAHA.108.192218.

23. Eigenbrodt ML, Rose KM, Couper DJ, Arnett DK, Smith R, Jones D. Orthostatic hypotension as a risk factor for stroke: the atherosclerosis risk in communities (ARIC) study, 1987-1996. Stroke. 2000;31(10):2307–13.

24. Fagard RH, Celis H, Thijs L, Staessen JA, Clement DL, De Buyzere ML, De Bacquer DA. Daytime and nighttime blood pressure as predictors of death and cause-specific cardiovascular events in hypertension. Hypertension. 2008;51(1):55–61.

25. Farnsworth TA, Heseltine D. The effect of postprandial hypotension on rehabilitation of the frail elderly with cerebrovascular disease. J Int Med Res. 1994;22(2):77–84.

26. Fedorowski A, Stavenow L, Hedblad B, Berglund G, Nilsson PM, Melander O. Orthostatic hypotension predicts all-cause mortality and coronary events in middle-aged individuals (The Malmo Preventive Project). Eur Heart J. 2010;31(1):85–91. https://doi.org/10.1093/eurheartj/ehp329.

27. Fedorowski A, Wahlstrand B, Hedner T, Melander O. Systolic and diastolic component of orthostatic hypotension and cardiovascular events in hypertensive patients: the Captopril Prevention Project. J Hypertens. 2014;32(1):75–81. https://doi.org/10.1097/HJH.0b013e328365cd59.

28. Feldstein C, Weder AB. Orthostatic hypotension: a common, serious and underrecognized problem in hospitalized patients. J Am Soc Hypertens. 2012;6(1):27–39. https://doi.org/10.1016/j.jash.2011.08.008.
29. Fisher AA, Davis MW, Srikusalanukul W, Budge MM. Postprandial hypotension predicts all-cause mortality in older, low-level care residents. J Am Geriatr Soc. 2005;53(8):1313–20.
30. García-Albea E, Cabrera-Valdivia F, Jiménez-Jiménez FJ, Tejeiro J, Vaquero A, Manzano L, Alvarez de Mon M. Unilateral carotid sinus hypersensitivity as a sign of occlusion of the internal carotid artery. Rev Neurol. 1999;29(4):390.
31. Geeganage C, Bath PM. Interventions for deliberately altering blood pressure in acute stroke. Cochrane Database Syst Rev. 2008;4:CD000039. https://doi.org/10.1002/14651858.CD000039.pub2.
32. Geeganage C, Bath PM. Vasoactive drugs for acute stroke. Cochrane Database Syst Rev. 2010;7:CD002839. https://doi.org/10.1002/14651858.CD002839.pub2.
33. Gong S, Lin C, Zhang D, Kong X, Chen J, Wang C, Li Z, Chen R, Sheng P, Dong Y, Hou L. Effects of intensive blood pressure reduction on acute intracerebral hemorrhage: a systematic review and meta-analysis. Sci Rep. 2017;7(1):10694.
34. Hemphill JC 3rd, Greenberg SM, Anderson CS, Becker K, Bendok BR, Cushman M, Fung GL, Goldstein JN, Macdonald RL, Mitchell PH, Scott PA, Selim MH, Woo D, American Heart Association Stroke Council; Council on Cardiovascular and Stroke Nursing, Council on Clinical Cardiology. Guidelines for the management of spontaneous intracerebral hemorrhage: a guideline for healthcare professionals from the American Heart Association/American Stroke Association. Stroke. 2015;46(7):2032–60. https://doi.org/10.1161/STR.0000000000000069.
35. Hermida RC, Ayala DE, Mojón A, Fernández JR. Influence of circadian time of hypertension treatment on cardiovascular risk: results of the MAPEC study. Chronobiol Int. 2010;27(8):1629–51. https://doi.org/10.3109/07420528.2010.510230.
36. Jansen RW, Lipsitz LA. Postprandial hypotension: epidemiology, pathophysiology, and clinical management. Ann Intern Med. 1995;122(4):286–95.
37. Juraschek SP, Daya N, Appel LJ, Miller ER 3rd, McEvoy JW, Matsushita K, Ballantyne CM, Selvin E. Orthostatic hypotension and risk of clinical and subclinical cardiovascular disease in middle-aged adults. J Am Heart Assoc. 2018;7(10) https://doi.org/10.1161/JAHA.118.008884. pii: e008884.
38. Kario K, Matsuo T, Kobayashi H, Imiya M, Matsuo M, Shimada K. Nocturnal fall of blood pressure and silent cerebrovascular damage in elderly hypertensive patients. Advanced silent cerebrovascular damage in extreme dippers. Hypertension. 1996;27(1):130–5.
39. Kario K, Pickering TG, Matsuo T, Hoshide S, Schwartz JE, Shimada K. Stroke prognosis and abnormal nocturnal blood pressure falls in older hypertensives. Hypertension. 2001;38(4):852–7.
40. Kario K, Shimada K, Pickering TG. Abnormal nocturnal blood pressure falls in elderly hypertension: clinical significance and determinants. J Cardiovasc Pharmacol. 2003;41(Suppl 1):S61–6.
41. Kjeldsen SE, Narkiewicz K, Burnier M. Oparil S4 The INTERSTROKE Study: hypertension is by far the most important modifiable risk factor for stroke. Blood Press. 2017;26(3):131–2. https://doi.org/10.1080/08037051.2017.1292456.
42. Kohara K, Jiang Y, Igase M, Takata Y, Fukuoka T, Okura T, Kitami Y, Hiwada K. Postprandial hypotension is associated with asymptomatic cerebrovascular damage in essential hypertensive patients. Hypertension. 1999;33(1 Pt 2):565–8.
43. Krajewski A, Freeman R, Ruthazer R, Kelley M, Lipsitz LA. Doppler assessment of the cerebral circulation during postprandial hypotension in the elderly. Transcranial J Am Geriatr Soc. 1993;41(1):19–24.
44. Kvistad CE, Logallo N, Oygarden H, Thomassen L, Waje-Andreassen U, Naess H. Elevated admission blood pressure and stroke severity in acute ischemic stroke: the Bergen NORSTROKE Study. Cerebrovasc Dis. 2013;36(5–6):351–4. https://doi.org/10.1159/000355685. Epub 2013 Oct 30.

45. Lai B, Jeng B, Vrongistinos K, Jung T. Post-exercise hypotensive responses following an acute bout of aquatic and overground treadmill walking in people post-stroke: a pilot study. Top Stroke Rehabil. 2015;22(3):231–8. https://doi.org/10.1179/1074935714Z.0000000016.

46. Li L, Yiin GS, Geraghty OC, Schulz UG, Kuker W, Mehta Z, Rothwell PM, Oxford Vascular Study. Incidence, outcome, risk factors, and long-term prognosis of cryptogenic transient ischaemic attack and ischaemic stroke: a population-based study. Lancet Neurol. 2015;14(9):903–13. https://doi.org/10.1016/S1474-4422(15)00132-5.

47. Liu Y, Yang Y, Jin H, Fan C, Lv P, Sun W, Peng Q, Zhao M, Jin DK, Wang J, Wong LKS, Anderson CS, Zheng L, Huang Y, ChinaQUEST (Quality Evaluation of Stroke Care and Treatment) Investigators. Discrepant relationships between admission blood pressure and mortality in different stroke subtypes. J Neurol Sci. 2017;383:47–51. https://doi.org/10.1016/j.jns.2017.09.032.

48. Low PA, Tomalia VA. Orthostatic hypotension: mechanisms, causes, management. J Clin Neurol. 2015;11(3):220–6. https://doi.org/10.3988/jcn.2015.11.3.220.

49. Low PA. Prevalence of orthostatic hypotension. Clin Auton Res. 2008;18(Suppl 1):8–13. https://doi.org/10.1007/s10286-007-1001-3.

50. Mangla R, Kolar B, Almast J, Ekholm SE. Border zone infarcts: pathophysiologic and imaging characteristics. Radiographics. 2011;31(5):1201–14. https://doi.org/10.1148/rg.315105014.

51. Martins AI, Sargento-Freitas J, Jesus-Ribeiro J, Correia I, Cardoso L, Gomes JP, Gonçalves M, Costa R, Silva F, Galego O, Nunes C, Beato-Coelho J, Varela R, Machado C, Rodrigues B, Santo GC, Cunha L. Blood pressure variability in acute ischemic stroke: the role of early recanalization. Eur Neurol. 2018;80(1–2):63–7. https://doi.org/10.1159/000492627.

52. Mattle HP, Kappeler L, Arnold M, Fischer U, Nedeltchev K, Remonda L, Jakob SM, Schroth G. Blood pressure and vessel recanalization in the first hours after ischemic stroke. Stroke. 2005;36(2):264–8.

53. Medow MS, Stewart JM, Sanyal S, Mumtaz A, Sica D, Frishman WH. Pathophysiology, diagnosis, and treatment of orthostatic hypotension and vasovagal syncope. Cardiol Rev. 2008;16(1):4–20.

54. Metzler M, Duerr S, Granata R, Krismer F, Robertson D, Wenning GK. Neurogenic orthostatic hypotension: pathophysiology, evaluation, and management. J Neurol. 2013;260(9):2212–9. https://doi.org/10.1007/s00415-012-6736-7.

55. Momjian-Mayor I, Baron JC. The pathophysiology of watershed infarction in internal carotid artery disease: review of cerebral perfusion studies. Stroke. 2005;36(3):567–77.

56. Mozaffarian D, Benjamin EJ, Go AS, Arnett DK, Blaha MJ, Cushman M, Das SR, de Ferranti S, Després JP, Fullerton HJ, Howard VJ, Huffman MD, Isasi CR, Jiménez MC, Judd SE, Kissela BM, Lichtman JH, Lisabeth LD, Liu S, Mackey RH, Magid DJ, McGuire DK, Mohler ER 3rd, Moy CS, Muntner P, Mussolino ME, Nasir K, Neumar RW, Nichol G, Palaniappan L, Pandey DK, Reeves MJ, Rodriguez CJ, Rosamond W, Sorlie PD, Stein J, Towfighi A, Turan TN, Virani SS, Woo D, Yeh RW, Turner MB, American Heart Association Statistics Committee; Stroke Statistics Subcommittee. Heart disease and stroke statistics-2016 update: a report from the American Heart Association. Circulation. 2016;133(4):e38–360.

57. Nguyen TAN, Ali Abdelhamid Y, Weinel LM, Hatzinikolas S, Kar P, Summers MJ, Phillips LK, Horowitz M, Jones KL, Deane AM. Postprandial hypotension in older survivors of critical illness. J Crit Care. 2018;45:20–6. https://doi.org/10.1016/j.jcrc.2018.01.012.

58. Novak V, Hu K, Desrochers L, Novak P, Caplan L, Lipsitz L, Selim M. Cerebral flow velocities during daily activities depend on blood pressure in patients with chronic ischemic infarctions. Stroke. 2010;41(1):61–6. https://doi.org/10.1161/STROKEAHA.109.565556.

59. O'Donnell MJ, Chin SL, Rangarajan S, Xavier D, Liu L, Zhang H, Rao-Melacini P, Zhang X, Pais P, Agapay S, Lopez-Jaramillo P, Damasceno A, Langhorne P, McQueen MJ, Rosengren A, Dehghan M, Hankey GJ, Dans AL, Elsayed A, Avezum A, Mondo C, Diener HC, Ryglewicz D, Czlonkowska A, Pogosova N, Weimar C, Iqbal R, Diaz R, Yusoff K, Yusufali A, Oguz A, Wang X, Penaherrera E, Lanas F, Ogah OS, Ogunniyi A, Iversen HK, Malaga G, Rumboldt Z, Oveisgharan S, Al Hussain F, Magazi D, Nilanont Y, Ferguson J, Pare G, Yusuf S,

INTERSTROKE investigators. Global and regional effects of potentially modifiable risk factors associated with acute stroke in 32 countries (INTERSTROKE): a case-control study. Lancet. 2016;388(10046):761–75.

60. Pandian JD, Wong AA, Lincoln DJ, Davis JP, Henderson RD, O'Sullivan JD, Read SJ. Circadian blood pressure variation after acute stroke. J Clin Neurosci. 2006;13(5):558–62. Epub 2006 May 5.

61. Park JH, Lee HS, Kim JH, Lee JH, Kim J, Choi SW. Reverse dipper and high night-time heart rate in acute stage of cerebral infarction are associated with increased mortality. J Stroke Cerebrovasc Dis. 2014;23(5):1171–6.

62. Pavelić A, Krbot Skorić M, Crnošija L, Habek M. Postprandial hypotension in neurological disorders: systematic review and meta-analysis. Clin Auton Res. 2017;27(4):263–71. https://doi.org/10.1007/s10286-017-0440-8.

63. Pierdomenico SD, Di Nicola M, Esposito AL, Di Mascio R, Ballone E, Lapenna D, Cuccurullo F. Prognostic value of different indices of blood pressure variability in hypertensive patients. Am J Hypertens. 2009;22(8):842–7. https://doi.org/10.1038/ajh.2009.103.

64. Pierdomenico SD, Pierdomenico AM, Coccina F, Lapenna D, Porreca E. Circadian blood pressure changes and cardiovascular risk in elderly-treated hypertensive patients. Hypertens Res. 2016;39(11):805–11. https://doi.org/10.1038/hr.2016.74.

65. Poon IO, Braun U. High prevalence of orthostatic hypotension and its correlation with potentially causative medications among elderly veterans. J Clin Pharm Ther. 2005;30(2):173–8.

66. Powers WJ, Rabinstein AA, Ackerson T, Adeoye OM, Bambakidis NC, Becker K, Biller J, Brown M, Demaerschalk BM, Hoh B, Jauch EC, Kidwell CS, Leslie-Mazwi TM, Ovbiagele B, Scott PA, Sheth KN, Southerland AM, Summers DV, Tirschwell DL, American Heart Association Stroke Council. 2018 guidelines for the early management of patients with acute ischemic stroke: a guideline for healthcare professionals from the American Heart Association/American Stroke Association. Stroke. 2018;49(3):e46–e110. https://doi.org/10.1161/STR.0000000000000158.

67. Rawlings AM, Juraschek SP, Heiss G, Hughes T, Meyer ML, Selvin E, Sharrett AR, Windham BG, Gottesman RF. Association of orthostatic hypotension with incident dementia, stroke, and cognitive decline. Neurology. 2018;91(8):e759–68. https://doi.org/10.1212/WNL.0000000000006027.

68. Regenhardt RW, Das AS, Stapleton CJ, Chandra RV, Rabinov JD, Patel AB, Hirsch JA, Leslie-Mazwi TM. Blood pressure and penumbral sustenance in stroke from large vessel occlusion. Front Neurol. 2017;8:317. https://doi.org/10.3389/fneur.2017.00317.

69. Reinprecht F, Axelsson J, Siennicki-Lantz A, Elmståhl S. Low nocturnal blood pressure is associated with reduced cerebral blood flow in the cohort "Men born in 1914". Int J Angiol. 2008;17(2):71–7.

70. Rodriguez J, Blaber AP, Kneihsl M, Trozic I, Ruedl R, Green DA, Broadbent J, Xu D, Rössler A, Hinghofer-Szalkay H, Fazekas F, Goswami N. Poststroke alterations in heart rate variability during orthostatic challenge. Medicine (Baltimore). 2017;96(14):e5989.

71. Romme JJ, van Dijk N, Boer KR, Dekker LR, Stam J, Reitsma JB, Wieling W. Influence of age and gender on the occurrence and presentation of reflex syncope. Clin Auton Res. 2008;18(3):127–33. https://doi.org/10.1007/s10286-008-0465-0.

72. Rose KM, Eigenbrodt ML, Biga RL, Couper DJ, Light KC, Sharrett AR, Heiss G. Orthostatic hypotension predicts mortality in middle-aged adults: the Atherosclerosis Risk In Communities (ARIC) Study. Circulation. 2006;114(7):630–6.

73. Ruzicka M, Edwards C, McCormick B, Hiremath S. Thus far and no further: should diastolic hypotension limit intensive blood pressure lowering? Curr Treat Options Cardiovasc Med. 2017;19(10):80. https://doi.org/10.1007/s11936-017-0577-8.

74. Sacco RL, Kasner SE, Broderick JP, Caplan LR, Connors JJ, Culebras A, Elkind MS, George MG, Hamdan AD, Higashida RT, Hoh BL, Janis LS, Kase CS, Kleindorfer DO, Lee JM, Moseley ME, Peterson ED, Turan TN, Valderrama AL, Vinters HV, American Heart Association Stroke Council, Council on Cardiovascular Surgery and Anesthesia, Council on

Cardiovascular Radiology and Intervention, Council on Cardiovascular and Stroke Nursing, Council on Epidemiology and Prevention; Council on Peripheral Vascular Disease, Council on Nutrition, Physical Activity and Metabolism. An updated definition of stroke for the 21st century: a statement for healthcare professionals from the American Heart Association/American Stroke Association. Stroke. 2013;44(7):2064–89.

75. Salles GF, Reboldi G, Fagard RH, Cardoso CR, Pierdomenico SD, Verdecchia P, Eguchi K, Kario K, Hoshide S, Polonia J, de la Sierra A, Hermida RC, Dolan E, O'Brien E, Roush GC, ABC-H Investigators. Prognostic effect of the nocturnal blood pressure fall in hypertensive patients: the ambulatory blood pressure collaboration in patients with hypertension (ABC-H) meta-analysis. Hypertension. 2016;67(4):693–700.

76. Sargento-Freitas J, Laranjinha I, Galego O, Rebelo-Ferreira A, Moura B, Correia M, Silva F, Machado C, Cordeiro G, Cunha L. Nocturnal blood pressure dipping in acute ischemic stroke. Acta Neurol Scand. 2015;132(5):323–8. https://doi.org/10.1111/ane.12402.

77. Savitz SI, Caplan LR. Vertebrobasilar disease. N Engl J Med. 2005;352(25):2618–26.

78. Schönenberger S, Uhlmann L, Ungerer M, Pfaff J, Nagel S, Klose C, Bendszus M, Wick W, Ringleb PA, Kieser M, Möhlenbruch MA, Bösel J. Association of blood pressure with short- and long-term functional outcome after stroke thrombectomy: post hoc analysis of the SIESTA Trial. Stroke. 2018;49(6):1451–6. https://doi.org/10.1161/STROKEAHA.117.019709.

79. Shi L, Xu S, Zheng J, Xu J, Zhang J. Blood pressure management for acute intracerebral hemorrhage: a meta-analysis. Sci Rep. 2017;7(1):14345. https://doi.org/10.1038/s41598-017-13111-x.

80. Steiner T, Al-Shahi Salman R, Beer R, Christensen H, Cordonnier C, Csiba L, Forsting M, Harnof S, Klijn CJ, Krieger D, Mendelow AD, Molina C, Montaner J, Overgaard K, Petersson J, Roine RO, Schmutzhard E, Schwerdtfeger K, Stapf C, Tatlisumak T, Thomas BM, Toni D, Unterberg A, Wagner M, European Stroke Organisation. European Stroke Organisation (ESO) guidelines for the management of spontaneous intracerebral hemorrhage. Int J Stroke. 2014;9(7):840–55. https://doi.org/10.1111/ijs.12309.

81. Tabara Y, Okada Y, Uetani E, Nagai T, Igase M, Kido T, Ochi N, Ohara M, Takita R, Kohara K, Miki T. Postprandial hypotension as a risk marker for asymptomatic lacunar infarction. J Hypertens. 2014;32(5):1084–90; discussion 1090. https://doi.org/10.1097/HJH.0000000000000150.

82. Thijs RD, Bloem BR, van Dijk JG. Falls, faints, fits and funny turns. J Neurol. 2009;256(2):155–67. https://doi.org/10.1007/s00415-009-0108-y.

83. Trahair LG, Horowitz M, Jones KL. Postprandial hypotension: a systematic review. Am Med Dir Assoc. 2014;15(6):394–409. https://doi.org/10.1016/j.jamda.2014.01.011.

84. Vemmos KN, Tsivgoulis G, Spengos K, Zakopoulos N, Synetos A, Manios E, Konstantopoulou P, Mavrikakis M. U-shaped relationship between mortality and admission blood pressure in patients with acute stroke. J Intern Med. 2004;255(2):257–65.

85. Verdecchia P, Angeli F, Mazzotta G, Garofoli M, Ramundo E, Gentile G, Ambrosio G, Reboldi G. Day-night dip and early-morning surge in blood pressure in hypertension: prognostic implications. Hypertension. 2012;60(1):34–42.

86. Verwoert GC, Mattace-Raso FU, Hofman A, Heeringa J, Stricker BH, Breteler MM, Witteman JC. Orthostatic hypotension and risk of cardiovascular disease in elderly people: the Rotterdam study. J Am Geriatr Soc. 2008;56(10):1816–20. https://doi.org/10.1111/j.1532-5415.2008.01946.x.

87. Wang A, Abramowicz AE. Endovascular thrombectomy in acute ischemic stroke: new treatment guide. Curr Opin Anaesthesiol. 2018;31(4):473–80. https://doi.org/10.1097/ACO.0000000000000621.

88. Whalin MK, Lopian S, Wyatt K, Sun CH, Nogueira RG, Glenn BA, Gershon RY, Gupta R. Dexmedetomidine: a safe alternative to general anesthesia for endovascular stroke treatment. J Neurointerv Surg. 2014;6(4):270–5. https://doi.org/10.1136/neurintsurg-2013-010773.

89. WHO. The global burden of disease: 2004 update. Geneva: WHO; 2008.
90. Wohlfahrt P, Krajcoviechova A, Jozifova M, Mayer O, Vanek J, Filipovsky J, Cifkova R. Low blood pressure during the acute period of ischemic stroke is associated with decreased survival. J Hypertens. 2015;33(2):339–45. https://doi.org/10.1097/HJH.0000000000000414.
91. Xin W, Mi S, Lin Z, Wang H, Wei W. Orthostatic hypotension and the risk of incidental cardiovascular diseases: a meta-analysis of prospective cohort studies. Prev Med. 2016;85:90–7. https://doi.org/10.1016/j.ypmed.2016.01.007.

Kannayiram Alagiakrishnan

Introduction

Parkinson's disease (PD) is one of the most common neurodegenerative disorder seen in the elderly. The median age of onset is between 60 and 65 years of age and peaks between 70 and 79 years old in most studies [1]. The incidence of PD is 1% of the population over the age of 60, and this increases to 5% over the age of 85. The main risk for PD is age [2, 3]. Severe disability is seen in 65% within 10 years of onset of disease. The costs associated with this disease are around $14 billion per year in the USA alone [4].

In PD, there is neuronal loss within the substantia nigra which projects to the putamen (the dopaminergic nigrostriatal pathway) and also to the noradrenergic neurons in locus coeruleus. Lewy body deposition is the main pathological change in PD. Lewy body is mainly composed of alpha-synuclein and belongs to the group of synucleinopathies. About 60% of nigrostriatal dopaminergic terminals are lost by the time the first clinical feature of PD seen [5]. Braak et al. proposed neuropathological staging of PD into six stages [6]. The cardinal clinical features are motor deficits, including tremor, rigidity and bradykinesia, traditionally associated with dopaminergic denervation in the substantia nigra [7]. There is however increased recognition of the importance of the disease-induced non-motor symptoms. Some of these non-motor abnormalities, including autonomic dysfunction, sleep disturbance, cognitive impairment and depression, which can precede the motor deficits by years or even decades [8].The basis for these non-motor deficits are still unclear, but it is suggested that many of them may be associated with alterations of non-dopaminergic neurotransmitter systems [9]. In particular, several in vivo and postmortem studies support the hypothesis that progressive alterations of the serotonergic system may contribute to a number of such non-motor symptoms [10].

K. Alagiakrishnan (✉)
Division of Geriatric Medicine, University of Alberta, Edmonton, AB, Canada

Motor Symptoms

The diagnosis of PD currently relies on the typical motor features. Rest tremor of the arms usually starts unilaterally with a pill-rolling character. Jaw tremors are seen sometimes, and head tremor is rare. Rigidity is the resistance of muscles to passive movement around a joint and lead type rigidity is commonly seen in PD. Bradykinesia is seen as slowness of movements as well as soft speech (hypophonia) and decreased facial expression (hypomimia). Other motor features of PD, include postural instability, gait initiation difficulties, freezing, progressively flexed posture, and dysphagia [11].

Non-motor Symptoms

Non-motor symptoms include disorders of sleep-wake cycle regulation, cognitive impairment, disorders of mood and affect, autonomic dysfunction, and sensory symptoms. Hyposmia or anosmia is present in 90% of patients with PD and may precede the onset of motor features. Autonomic dysfunction in PD encompasses bladder, bowel, and sexual dysfunction, as well as cardiovascular complications such as postural hypotension [12]. Cardiovascular autonomic dysfunction is common in PD, causing labile hypertension, orthostatic hypotension, and postprandial hypotension [13]. Typical Parkinson's disease progresses clinically, through several stages (prodrome, early stage, mid-stage, and advanced PD).

Atypical Parkinsonism or Parkinsonism Plus Syndrome

Parkinson plus syndrome include progressive supranuclear palsy (PSP), multiple system atrophy (MSA), and cortico-basal degeneration (CBD).

PSP
The prevalence varies from 1 to 6.5 per 100,000 [14]. PSP progresses much faster, causes more severe symptoms, responds very poorly to Parkinson's medication, and has a significantly reduced life expectancy. Different clinical phenotypes of PSP has been described. Classic PSP or otherwise known as Steele-Richardson-Olszewski syndrome accounts for 50% of patients. It is characterized by a symmetric akinetic rigid syndrome, vertical supranuclear gaze palsy, frontal deficits, prominent postural instability, and falls. Another phenotype PSP-parkinsonism is present in 30% of those with PSP. It is characterized by an asymmetric onset of tremor and moderate initial therapeutic response to levodopa. The earliest and most disabling symptom of PSP is usually gait and balance problems. A retrospective study by Williams et al. showed the average period from the onset of symptoms to the first fall in PSP is 16.8 months, as compared to 108 months in PD, 40.8 months in vascular Parkinsonism, and 42 months in MSA [15]. Ondo et al., in their case-control study used computerized posturography, showed that balance impairment in PSP is different from that PD. In contrast to the short and shuffling

steps, stooped posture, narrow base, flexed knees, and turning en bloc typically seen in PD, PSP patients have a stiff and broad-based gait, with a tendency to have their knees and trunk extended and arms slightly abducted as well as pivot turning has been observed [16].

PSP patients may complain of blurred vision, diplopia, and eye irritation. Decrease in blink rate, apraxia of eyelid opening, limitation or absence of convergence are seen [17]. Diminished vertical saccades elicited with the optokinetic (OKN) flag may be the earliest oculomotor sign of PSP [18]. Some patients may have a procerus sign which is due to a sustained contraction of the procerus muscle, and consists of a facial expression with astonished, worried, and reptile-like features [19]. Cardiovascular autonomic dysfunction is more commonly seen in PSP than in PD [20].

MSA

It is a progressive alpha-synucleinopathy neurodegenerative disease involving the basal ganglia, the cerebellum, and the brain stem. Variable combinations of Parkinsonism, autonomic failure, cerebellar ataxia, and pyramidal symptoms are seen [21].

Two major motor presentations, MSA-P subtype and MSA-C subtype, can be distinguished. MSA-associated Parkinsonism is dominated by progressive akinesia and rigidity and postural instability whereas tremor is less common than in idiopathic PD. The cerebellar disorder of MSA is composed of gait ataxia, limb kinetic ataxia, and scanning dysarthria, as well as cerebellar oculomotor disturbances. Autonomic failure develops in virtually all patients with MSA and orthostatic hypotension is present in two-thirds of patients [22]. Currently, there is no effective therapy in MSA. Symptomatic treatment is largely restricted to treat Parkinsonism and dysautonomia clinical symptoms. Parkinsonism in MSA responds poorly to levodopa, and cerebellar ataxia is unresponsive to drug treatment.

CBD

In CBD, in addition to Parkinsonism features, cortical sensory deficits and alien-limb phenomenon are seen. Tremor is rare and dystonias can be seen. Behavioral changes, executive dysfunction, visuospatial deficits, and language problems like agrammatism may be observed in CBD subjects [23, 24].

Diagnosis The diagnosis of Parkinsonism and Parkinsonism plus syndromes is clinical. Currently there is no single test or biomarker that can accurately diagnose or refute the presence of PD [25]. MRI of the brain midsagittal view in PSP may show "hummingbird sign" or "penguin sign," which is due to the atrophy of the most rostral midbrain tegmentum, pontine base, and cerebellum, which appear to correlate with the head, body, and wing of these birds. Other feature seen in MRI is the "morning glory sign," which is due to midbrain atrophy with concavity of the lateral margin of the midbrain tegmentum, resembling the morning glory flower [26]. Fluorodeoxyglucose PET (FDG-PET) scan shows glucose hypometabolism in the midbrain and also decreased metabolic activity in the caudate, putamen, and prefrontal cortex in PSP patients [27].

Hypotensive Syndromes in Parkinson's Disease

Orthostatic Hypotension and Parkinson's Disease

Orthostatic hypotension (OH) is a common non-motor clinical feature of Parkinson's disease. A systematic review showed prevalence of OH in PD of about 30% [28]. Roughly one-third of PD patients with OH did not have orthostatic symptoms. Functional impairments and falls are seen similarly both in subjects with asymptomatic and symptomatic OH and also with severe OH [29]. A retrospective study had shown OH can increase the healthcare cost by $ 15,000 per patient per year and can also increase in healthcare utilization due to falls and neuropsychiatric symptoms. So screening of OH in Parkinson's disease is ideal [30]. Autonomic symptoms began 3 years before motor deficits and a case report showed neurogenic orthostatic hypotension as the initial feature of Parkinson's disease [31]. In atypical Parkinsonism patients, symptomatic OH is seen in up to 27% and in multiple system atrophy (MSA) up to 80% [32].OH may gradually and critically impact quality of life in Parkinsonian patients [33]. OH and supine hypertension (SH) is also seen in these subjects. The mechanism for SH associated with OH in patients with PD is not definitely known and possibly due to baroreflex failure [34].

Postprandial Hypotension and Parkinson's Disease

In 1977 Seyer Hansen first described postprandial hypotension (PPH) in a patient with PD [35]. Few studies in PD patients showed PPH was found to be correlated to OH in these subjects [36, 37]. A study by Umehara et al. showed in elderly with de novo PD the presence of severe dysnomia, constipation, OH, and preprandial hypertension at rest was associated with PPH [38]. In PD subjects, systemic sympathetic denervation and baroreflex failure contribute to both PPH and OH [39]. A study on Mehagnoul-Scripper et al. showed treatment with 125-mg b.i.d. doses of levodopa/benserazide did not significantly aggravate orthostatic or postprandial hypotension [40].

Carotid Sinus Syndrome (CSS) and Parkinson's Disease

CSS has two types, cardioinhibitory and vasodepressor types, and vasodepressor type is associated with hypotension. There appears to be a high prevalence of carotid sinus hypersensitivity (CSH) in patients with Lewy body dementia (DLB) [41, 42].

Exercise-Induced Hypotension and Parkinson's Disease

Exercise-induced hypotension can occur in Parkinson's disease patients with autonomic failure with the magnitude of the exercise response being related to the severity of autonomic dysfunction. Exercise does not appear to worsen OH in Parkinson's patients [43].

Vasovagal Syncope (VVS) and Parkinson's Disease

VVS starting in old age appears to be an expression of neurological or cardiovascular diseases [44]. Neurogenic orthostatic hypotension due to typical and atypical PD can often be differentiated from vasovagal syncope by its differing hemodynamic patterns during tilt table test and differing clinical characteristics [45].

Nocturnal Hypotension and Parkinson's Disease

OH in PD can also influence nocturnal blood pressure patterns. A study assessed the effect of OH with abnormal nocturnal BP profiles on dementia in PD. Among patients with OH, high prevalence of dementia is seen in extreme dippers (67%), when compared with dippers (13%) and non-dippers (30%) [46].

Mechanisms of Hypotensive Syndromes in PD

In all PD patients, nigrostriatal dopamine depletion is seen. In addition with patient's having hypotensive syndromes, noradrenergic denervation in both cardiac and extracardiac regions and arterial baroreflex failure are also seen. This pathophysiologic cause could also induce postprandial hypotension, instability of blood pressure in exercise-induced hypotension. Baroreflex failure involves both cardiovagal and sympathoneural limbs [47]. Positron emission tomography (PET) scanning showed that this denervation is profound in the heart but also could be detected in extracardiac organs such as the renal cortex and thyroid gland [48]. Synuclein accumulation in intraneural Lewy bodies of the limbic cortex, frontal neocortical areas, and the peripheral autonomic dysfunction can explain the more cognitive decline observed in PD patients suffering from OH [49].

Gastrointestinal function plays a role in the pathophysiology of PPH in PD. Braak et al. showed the earliest appearance of Lewy body pathology was seen in the myenteric plexus in the gut and the dorsal motor nucleus in the lower medulla in alpha-synuclein staining studies [50]. In PD, gastroparesis and slowed bowel movement can contribute to PPH by dysfunction of the enteric autonomic nervous system [51]. Insufficient postprandial sympathetic activation may also contribute to PPH in PD [39, 52] (Table 15.1).

Table 15.1 Mechanisms of hypotensive syndromes in PD

Autonomic dysfunction
Abnormal cerebral vasomotor reactivity
Baroreflex failure
Cardiac and extracardiac sympathetic denervation
Gastroparesis and slowed intestinal function

Table 15.2 Autonomic function tests in PD

Cardiovascular
24 hour Ambulatory Blood pressure:
OH, PPH, Non- dipping status and supine hypertension
Electrocardiography monitoring:
Heart rate response to Valsalva maneuver and deep breathing
Central
Cerebral vasomotor reactivity by transcranial Doppler

Testing for Central Autonomic Failure

Both central and peripheral autonomic failure can cause OH. In a small study evaluation of cerebral vasomotor reactivity by transcranial Doppler in PD subjects was shown to assist in the early diagnosis of cerebral autonomic dysfunction [53]. Other clinical features and tests which help to differentiate central (preganglionic) from peripheral autonomic failure (postganglionic) include normal auditory function, normal cardiac SNS innervations testing using 123I-MIBG (m-iodobenzylguanidine) scan, and quantitative sudomotor axonal reflex testing [45] (Table 15.2).

Management of Hypotensive Syndromes in PD

Since autonomic dysfunction is commonly seen in Parkinson's disease, management of OH is challenging [54]. In addition the medications used to treat PD may also cause associated hypotensive effect. PD-related medications such as selegiline and dopamine agonists also contribute to the OH. Levodopa has vasodilative effects via the renal and splanchnic vasculature, and it can cause or worsen OH. Withdrawal of selegiline suppresses the orthostatic blood pressure reaction in advanced PD patients [55–59]. Dopaminergic medications in large doses are associated with severity of OH [60, 61].

Non-pharmacological Therapies

OH in Parkinson's disease can be treated with sufficient fluid intake. Ingestion of half a litre of water in less than 5 minutes substantially raises blood pressure in MSA subjects with autonomic failure [62]. Other strategies like increasing salt intake and using compression stockings can be useful. If the patient has associated PPH, frequent smaller meals rather than three large meals can be helpful. If PPH occurs, avoid large meals and alcohol, increase salt intake if no contraindication and avoid straining stool.

Pharmacological Therapies

Midodrine showed significant benefit in randomized placebo-controlled trials in patients with OH [63]. Last dose should not be given no later than mid-afternoon to prevent supine hypertension at night. Other medications one can try are fludrocortisone and pyridostigmine. Fludrocortisone can cause hypokalemia, pedal edema, and supine hypertension. Pyridostigmine may increase drooling and urinary frequency. Droxidopa, the norepinephrine precursor l-threo-dihydroxyphenylserine (l-threo-DOPS), has been shown to be effective in placebo-controlled trials including patients with MSA [64]. Reassess antihypertensive agents, and see whether they contribute to hypotensive syndromes.

The goal of management of orthostatic hypotension is to raise the patient's standing blood pressure without also raising his or her supine blood pressure, and specifically to reduce orthostatic symptoms, increase the time the patient can stand, and improve his or her ability to perform daily activities. No specific treatment is currently available that achieves all these goals, and drugs alone are never completely adequate. Neurogenic orthostatic hypotension, postprandial hypotension, and supine hypertension can co-exist, and blood pressure lability is seen in PD with autonomic failure [65, 66]. Sleeping with the head of the bed elevated by 6–9 inches overnight time has been shown to decrease nocturnal supine hypertension and diuresis, and reduce day time OH episodes by increasing vasomotor tone [67]. Pyridostigmine may reduce the postural drop in blood pressure without causing supine hypertension [68]. Another drug which has been shown useful in OH due to PD and approved by FDA is droxidopa [69]. A meta-analysis showed droxidopa in neurogenic orthostatic hypotension subjects was well tolerated and also effective in reducing the OH symptoms without increasing the risk of supine hypertension [70].

Conclusions Hypotensive syndromes are commonly seen in PD with autonomic dysfunction. Management of these hypotensive syndromes is challenging. Despite the pharmacological options, treatment of symptomatic hypotensive syndromes in PD remains suboptimal, and future research is needed to address the challenges of management.

References

1. Ascherio A, Schwarzschild MA. The epidemiology of Parkinson's disease: risk factors and prevention. Lancet Neurol. 2016;15(12):1257–72.
2. Reeve A, Simcox E, Turnbull D. Ageing and Parkinson's disease: why is advancing age the biggest risk factor? Ageing Res Rev. 2014;14(100):19–30.
3. Politis M, Wu K, Molloy S, et al. Parkinson's disease symptoms: the patient's perspective. Mov Disord. 2010;25(11):1646–51.
4. Kowal SL, Dall TM, Chakrabarti R, et al. The current and projected economic burden of Parkinson's disease in the United States. Mov Disord. 2013;28:311–8.
5. Dickson DW, Braak H, Duda JE, et al. Neuropathological assessment of Parkinson's disease: refining the diagnostic criteria. Lancet Neurol. 2009;8(12):1150–7.
6. Braak H, Del Tredic K, Rüb U, et al. Staging of brain pathology related to sporadic Parkinson's disease. Neurobiol Aging. 2003;24:197–211.
7. Stoessl AJ, Vaillancourt D, Spraker M. Neuroimaging in Parkinson's disease: from pathology to diagnosis. Parkinsonism Relat Disord. 2012;18(Suppl. 1):S55–9.
8. Schrag A, Horsfall L, Walters K, et al. Prediagnostic presentations of Parkinson's disease in primary care: a case-control study. Lancet Neurol. 2015;14;57–64.

9. Stoessl AJ. Functional imaging studies of non-motoric manifestations of Parkinson's disease. Parkinsonism Relat Disord. 2009;15:S13–6.
10. Politis M, Loane C. Serotonergic dysfunction in Parkinson's disease and its relevance to disability. Sci World J. 2011;11:1726–34.
11. Hess CW, Okun MS. Diagnosing Parkinson disease. Neurol Contin. 2016;22(4):1047–63.
12. Goldstein DS. Orthostatic hypotension as an early finding in Parkinson's disease. Clin Auton Res. 2006;16:46–54.
13. Schapira AHV, Chaudhuri KR, Jenner P. Non-motor features of Parkinson disease. Nat Rev Neurosci. 2017;18(7):435–50.
14. Nath U, Ben-Shlomo Y, Thomson RG, et al. The prevalence of progressive supranuclear palsy (Steele–Richardson–Olszewski syndrome) in the UK. Brain. 2001;124(7):1438–49.
15. Williams DR, Watt HC, Lees AJ. Predictors of falls and fractures in bradykinetic rigid syndromes: a retrospective study. J Neurol Neurosurg Psychiatry. 2006;77(4):468–73.
16. Ondo W, Warrior D, Overby A, et al. Computerized posturography analysis of progressive supranuclear palsy: a case–control comparison with Parkinson's disease and healthy controls. Arch Neurol. 2000;57(10):1464–9.
17. Jankovic J. Apraxia of lid opening. Mov Disord. 1995;10(5):686–7.
18. Garbutt S, Riley DE, Kumar AN, Han Y, Harwood MR, Leigh RJ. Abnormalities of optokinetic nystagmus in progressive supranuclear palsy. J Neurol Neurosurg Psychiatry. 2004;75(10):1386–94.
19. Romano S, Colosimo C. Procerus sign in progressive supranuclear palsy. Neurology. 2001;57(10):1928.
20. Schmidt C, Herting B, Prieur S, et al. Autonomic dysfunction in patients with progressive supranuclear palsy. Mov Disord. 2008;23(14):2083–9.
21. Wenning GK, Colosimo C, Geser F, et al. Multiple system atrophy. Lancet Neurol. 2004;3:93–103.
22. Kollensperger M, Wenning GK. Assessing disease progression with MRI in atypical parkinsonian disorders. Mov Disord. 2009;24(Suppl 2):S699–702.
23. Armstrong MJ, Litvan I, Lang AE, et al. Criteria for the diagnosis of corticobasal degeneration. Neurology. 2013;80:496–503.
24. Murray R, Neumann M, Forman MS, et al. Cognitive and motor assessment in autopsy-proven corticobasal degeneration. Neurology. 2007;68:1274–83.
25. Poewe W, Seppi K, Tanner CM, et al. Parkinson disease. Nat Rev Dis Primers. 2017;3:17013.
26. Oba H, Yagishita A, Terada H, et al. New and reliable MRI diagnosis for progressive supranuclear palsy. Neurology. 2005;64(12):2050–5.
27. Mishina M, Ishii K, Mitani K, et al. Midbrain hypometabolism as early diagnostic sign for progressive supranuclear palsy. Acta Neurol Scand. 2004;110(2):128–35.
28. Velseboer DC, de Haan RJ, Wieling W, et al. Prevalence of orthostatic hypotension in Parkinson's disease: a systematic review and meta- analysis. Park Relat Disord. 2011;17:724–9.
29. Merolaa A, Romagnolob A, Rossoa M. Orthostatic hypotension in Parkinson's disease: does it matter if asymptomatic? Park Relat Disord. 2016;33:65–71.
30. Merola A, Sawyer RP, Artusi CA. Orthostatic hypotension in Parkinson disease: impact on health care utilization. Parkinsonism Relat Disord. 2018;47:45–9.
31. Milazzo V, Di Stefano C, Servo S, et al. Neurogenic orthostatic hypotension as the initial feature of Parkinson disease. Clin Auton Res. 2012;22(4):203–6.
32. Ha AD, Brown CH, York MK, et al. The prevalence of symptomatic orthostatic hypotension in patients with Parkinson's disease and atypical parkinsonism. Parkinsonism Relat Disord. 2011;17(8):625–8.
33. Gallagher DA, Lees AJ, Schrag A. What are the most important nonmotor symptoms in patients with Parkinson's disease and are we missing them? Mov Disord. 2010;25(15):2493–500.
34. Sharabi Y, Goldstein DS. Mechanisms of orthostatic hypotension and supine hypertension in Parkinson disease. J Neurol Sci. 2011;310:123–8.
35. Seyer- Hansen K. Postprandial hypotension. Br Med J. 1977;2:1262.

36. Micieli G, Martignoni E, Cavallini A, et al. Postprandial and orthostatic hypotension in Parkinson's disease. Neurology. 1987;37:386–93.
37. Loew F, Gauthey L, Koerffy A, et al. Postprandial hypotension and orthostatic blood pressure responses in elderly Parkinson's disease patients. J Hypertens. 1995;13:1291–7.
38. Umehara T, Nakahara A, Matsuno H, et al. Predictors of postprandial hypotension in elderly patients with de novo Parkinson's Disease. J Neural Transm. 2016;122:1331–9.
39. Umehara T, Toyoda C, Oka H. Postprandial hypotension in de novo Parkinson's disease: a comparison with orthostatic hypotension. Parkinsonism Relat Disord. 2014;20:573–7.
40. Mehagnoul-Schipper DJ, Boerman RH, Hoefnagels WH, et al. Effect of levodopa on orthostatic and postprandial hypotension in elderly Parkinsonian patients. J Gerontol. 2001;A 56:M749–55.
41. Ballard C, Shaw F, McKeith I, et al. High prevalence of neurovascular instability in neurodegenerative dementias. Neurology. 1998;51:1760–2.
42. Kenny RA, Shaw FE, O'Brien JT, et al. Carotid sinus syndrome is common in dementia with Lewy bodies and correlates with deep white matter lesions. J Neurol Neurosurg Psychiatr. 2004;75(7):966–71.
43. Low DA, Vichayanrat E, Iodice V, et al. Exercise hemodynamics in Parkinson's disease and autonomic dysfunction. Parkinsonism Relat Disord. 2014;20(5):549–53.
44. Alboni P, Brignole M, Degli Uberti EC. Is vasovagal syncope a disease? Europace. 2007;9(2):83–7.
45. Nwazue VC, Raj SR. Confounders of Vasovagal syncope: orthostatic hypotension. Cardiol Clin. 2013;31(1):89–100.
46. Tanaka R, Shimo Y, Yamashiro K, et al. Association between abnormal nocturnal blood pressure profile and dementia in Parkinson's disease. Parkinsonism Relat Disord. 2018;46:24–9.
47. Jain S, Goldstein DS. Cardiovascular dysautonomia in Parkinson disease: from pathophysiology to pathogenesis. Neurobiol Dis. 2012;46(3):572–80.
48. Tipre DN, Goldstein DS. Cardiac and extracardiac sympathetic denervation in Parkinson's disease with orthostatic hypotension and in pure autonomic failure. J Nucl Med. 2005;46(11):1775–81.
49. Poewe W. Dysautonomia and cognitive dysfunction in Parkinson's disease. Mov Disord. 2007;22(Suppl 17):S374–8.
50. Braak H, Del Tredict K, Ru U, et al. Staging of brain pathology related to sporadic Parkinson disease. Neurobiol Aging. 2003;24:197–211.
51. Pfeiffer RF. Gastrointestinal dysfunction in Parkinson's disease. Lancet Neurol. 2001;2:107–16.
52. Hirayama M, Watanabe H, Koike Y, et al. Postprandial hypotension hemodynamic differences between multiple system atrophy and peripheral autonomic neuropathy. J Auton Nerv Syst. 1993;43:1–6.
53. Zamani B, Mehrabani M, Fereshtehnejad SM, et al. Evaluation of cerebral vasomotor reactivity in Parkinson's disease: is there any association with orthostatic hypotension? Clin Neurol Neurosurg. 2011;113(5):368–72.
54. Espay AJ, Lewitt PA, Hauser RA, et al. Neurogenic orthostatic hypotension and supine hypertension in Parkinson's disease and related synucleinopathies: prioritisation of treatment targets. Lancet Neurol. 2016;15:954.
55. Kujawa K, Leurgans S, Raman R, et al. Acute orthostatic hypotension when starting dopamine agonists in Parkinson's disease. Arch Neurol. 2000;57:1461–3.
56. Pursiainen V, Korpelainen TJ, Haapaniemi HT, et al. Selegiline and blood pressure in patients with Parkinson's disease. Acta Neurol Scand. 2007;115(2):104–8.
57. Haapaniemi TH, Kallio MA, Korpelainen JT, et al. Levodopa, bromocriptine and selegiline modify cardiovascular responses in Parkinson's disease. J Neurol. 2000;247(11):868–74.
58. Jankovic J, Stacy M. Medical management of levodopa-associated motor complications in patients with Parkinson's disease. CNS Drugs. 2007;21(8):677–92.
59. Mosnaim AD, Abiola R, Wolf ME, et al. Etiology and risk factors for developing orthostatic hypotension. Am J Ther. 2010;17(1):86–91.

60. Senard JM, Rai S, Lapeyre- Mestre M, et al. Prevalence of orthostatic hypotension in Parkinson's disease. J Neurol Neurosurg Psychiatry. 1997;63:584–9.
61. Allcock LM, Kenny RA, Burn DJ. Clinical phenotypes of subjects with Parkinson's disease and orthostatic hypotension: autonomic symptom and demographic comparison. Mov Disord. 2006;21:1851–5.
62. Young TM, Mathias CJ. The effects of water ingestion on orthostatic hypotension in two groups of chronic autonomic failure: multiple system atrophy and pure autonomic failure. J Neurol Neurosurg Psychiatry. 2004;75:1737–41.
63. Low PA, Gilden JL, Freeman R, et al. Efficacy of midodrine vs placebo in neurogenic orthostatic hypotension. A randomized, double-blind multicenter study. Midodrine Study Group. JAMA. 1997;277:1046–51.
64. Mathias CJ, Senard JM, Braune S, et al. L-Threo-dihydroxyphenylserine (l-threo-DOPS; droxidopa) in the management of neurogenic orthostatic hypotension: a multi-national, multi-center, dose-ranging study in multiple system atrophy and pure autonomic failure. Clin Auton Res. 2001;11:235–42.
65. Shibao C, Gamboa A, Diedrich A, et al. Management of hypertension in the setting of autonomic failure: a pathophysiological approach. Hypertension. 2005;45(4):469–76.
66. Pathak A, Senard JM. Blood pressure disorders during Parkinson's disease: epidemiology, pathophysiology and management. Expert Rev Neurother. 2006;6(8):1173–80.
67. Fan CW, Walsh C, Cunnigham CJ. The effect of sleeping with the head of the bed elevated six inches on elderly patients with orthostatic hypotension: an open randomized controlled trial. Age Ageing. 2011;40:187.
68. Singer W, Sandroni P, Opfer-Gehrking TL, et al. Pyridostigmine treatment trial in neurogenic orthostatic hypotension. Arch Neurol. 2006;63(4):513–8.
69. Isaacson SH, Skettini J. Neurogenic orthostatic hypotension in Parkinson's disease: evaluation, management, and emerging role of droxidopa. Vasc Health Risk Manag. 2014;10:169–76.
70. Victoria S, Julia LN, Maw Pin T, et al. Droxidopa for orthostatic hypotension: a systematic review and meta-analysis. J Hypertens. 2016;34(10):1933–41.

Kannayiram Alagiakrishnan

Introduction

Falls are defined as unintentionally coming to rest on the ground or a lower surface. More than one-third of adults age 65 or older fall each year. Seniors are one of the fastest growing population groups in the world. In simple terms, more ageing population equals more falls. Falls are the most common cause of injuries to older adults. The annual incidence of falls in patients over 65 years of age who live independently is approximately 25% but rises to 50% in patients over 80 years of age [1].

Falls occur in 30% of community-dwelling older persons [2–4]. Falls are 3 times more frequent in persons living in long-term care compared to those in the community [5]. Not surprisingly, given their widespread prevalence, falls also represent a major healthcare cost. In the United States, the total cost of falls injuries in 1994 for adults aged 65 years and older was estimated at $20.2 billion [6], whereas in 2015, the medical cost of falls in the United States was approximately $50 billion [7] and the cost has risen sharply in the two decades.

One-third of patients with confirmed falls may not recall falling [8]. It is a common cause of morbidity and the leading cause of nonfatal injuries and trauma-related hospitalizations. Falls are directly accountable for 40% of all elderly admissions to nursing homes or long-term care facilities [9]. Study has cited that injuries occur in up to 60% of falls [10]. Another common but often undetected consequence of fall is "fear of falling". Fear of falling has been identified in 25% of older people [11–13]. In the elderly, falls result in significant loss of confidence, fear of falling as well as loss of independence and increased likelihood of institutionalization. Falls are one of the top five sentinel events for hospitals, long-term care and home care agencies [14, 15].

Many risk factors have been identified for falls in older people. Epidemiological studies had documented the risk factors associated with falls in the community.

K. Alagiakrishnan (✉)
Division of Geriatric Medicine, University of Alberta, Edmonton, AB, Canada

© Springer Nature Switzerland AG 2020
K. Alagiakrishnan, M. Banach (eds.), *Hypotensive Syndromes in Geriatric Patients*, https://doi.org/10.1007/978-3-030-30332-7_16

These risks can be classified as intrinsic or host-related factors, extrinsic or environmental-/situational-related factors and behavioural risk factors. Intrinsic factors are medications, age-related changes in the balance systems, decreased vision, postural hypotension and urinary incontinence. Extrinsic factors include circumstances contributing to falls risk such as uneven pavement, slippery surfaces and poor lighting. Behaviour-related risk factors are hurrying, risk taking, physical inactivity and fear of falling. Many falls are due to a combination of intrinsic, extrinsic and behavioural factors. Falls prevention programs target at all these factors [16, 17].

Falls are responsible for a significant number of accidental deaths and traumatic injuries among the elderly. Among Canadian seniors aged 65 and older, falls accounted for 57% of deaths due to injuries among females and 36% among males [18]. Falls account for 70% of accidental deaths in those over 75 years of age [19]. Low systolic blood pressure increases the risk of falls in older persons and those with diabetes mellitus [20, 21]. Orthostatic hypotension has been associated with falls [22–24]. Postprandial hypotension is a common cause of falls in older persons and diabetics with autonomic neuropathy [25]. By treating these syndromes, there may be a possibility to prevent falls [26, 27]. In this chapter, how hypotensive syndromes as a single condition or in combination with other conditions play a role in falls has been discussed.

Mechanisms of Falls in Hypotensive Syndromes

The main mechanisms that cause falls in hypotensive syndromes could be due to syncope or neurocardiovascular or neuroautonomic instability. Hypotensive syndromes lead to cerebral hypoperfusion especially in those with a reset cerebral autoregulation and can cause falls [28]. Syncope commonly defined as a transient loss of consciousness could also be due to structural and arrhythmic cardiac causes, hypoglycaemia, seizures and transient ischemic attacks [29]. Table 16.1 shows the syncopal and non-syncopal causes of falls.

Neurocardiovascular instability (NCVI) refers to abnormal neural control of the cardiovascular system characterized by hypotension and heart rate changes which

Table 16.1 Syncopal and non-syncopal causes of falls

Syncope	Non-syncope
Vasovagal, carotid sinus, situational, drug- induced	Cataplexy
Autonomic failure- OH, PPH, PEH	Drop attacks
Cardiac causes- cardiac arrythmias, conduction disorders, cardiac pulmonary diseases- valvular diseases, ischemic heart disease, pulmonary embolism	Pyschogenic pseudo syncope
Cerebro vascular disease- like vascular steal syndromes, transient ischemic attacks	Transient ischemic attacks of carotid and vertebro basilar origin
Epilepsy-grand mal	Epilepsy-petit mal
Metabolic conditions like severe hypoglycaemia	Mild hypoglycaemia

plays a role in falls. Different hypotensive syndromes that characterize NCVI or neuroautonomic instability include postural hypotension, carotid sinus hypersensitivity, postprandial hypotension, exercise-related hypotension and vasovagal syncope. Autonomic dysfunction plays a major role in NCVI [30].

Different Hypotensive Syndromes and Their Association with Falls

Orthostatic Hypotension (OH) and Falls

The elderly of Boston study showed in hypertensive subjects that an asymptomatic systolic BP drop ≥20 mmHg in 1 minute of standing was predictive of falls [31]. In another study with nursing home residents, an association was shown between OH and previous recurrent falls [32]. In a prospective study by Menant JC et al., about 40% of the elderly subjects with unexplained falls had received previous diagnoses of orthostatic hypotension [33]. In a systematic review by Jansen S et al., the association between falls and orthostatic hypotension (OH) was ambivalent. This was attributed to the varied quality of reviewed studies which employed several different assessment methods to detect OH, inadequate details to enable adjustment for relevant confounders and sample populations which varied in size, most of which were convenience samples [34]. *Finucane et al. showed in the recent Irish Longitudinal Cohort Study on Ageing (TILDA) that OH was associated with increased relative risk of unexplained falls (RR 1.52, 95% CI 1.03–2.26) and was associated with all-cause falls (RR 1.40, 95% CI 1.01–1.96)* [35]. *This study also showed significantly increased risk of falls in those with sustained but not initial OH.* Although the Finucane paper emphasized the importance of beat-to-beat BP measurements to detect impaired orthostatic BP recovery as a risk factor for falls, this technology is not available in most clinical practices.

A recent prospective study also showed conventional methods of measuring blood pressure (BP) changes were too imprecise and the OH, defined according to 2011 criteria, was associated with falls. Using the 1996 consensus criteria (systolic/diastolic drop of >20/10 mmHg upon standing) there was no increased risk of falls [36], but when the 2011 consensus criteria were used (which includes updated criteria for initial OH and OH in the presence of hypertension) [37] there was a strong association between OH and falls (odds ratio 10.299, 95% confidence interval [95% CI]: 1.703–61.43, $P = 0.011$) and time to first fall (hazard ratio(HR) 3.017, 95% CI: 1.291–7.050, $P = 0.011$) [38]. Hartog et al. showed in the meta-analysis of prospective observational studies a significant relationship between OH and time to first fall incident (HR 1.52, 95% CI 1.23–1.88) [39].

It seems likely that orthostatic hypotension (OH) is a risk factor for falls. Beat to beat BP measurement, diagnostic criteria may influence the association between OH and falls. OH can cause ischemic damage to watershed regions of the brain. This damage manifests as white matter hyperintensities on brain imaging and is known to be associated with slow gait and falls [40, 41]. Adequate treatment of hypertension was shown to ameliorate OH and may prevent falls [42].

Postprandial Hypotension (PPH) and Falls

PPH is a drop in the systolic blood pressure after eating. Some of the common manifestations of PPH are dizziness, light-headedness and falls [43]. A study has shown PPH was associated with unexplained syncope [44]. Low postprandial systolic BP has been found in research studies, with subjects who has experienced falls [45, 46]. PPH can be treated with α-1-glucosidase inhibitors (acarbose or miglitol), which increase glucagon like peptide-1 and slow gastric emptying [25–27].

Carotid Sinus Hypersensitivity (CSH), Vasovagal Syncope (VVS) and Falls

CSH, VVS and OH are conditions that had been shown to co-exist in older subjects with falls [29]. Tan MP et al. in their case-control study found diagnoses of OH and VVS commonly co-exist in subjects with CSH and can lead to syncope and drop attacks [47].

Post-exercise Hypotension and Falls

Post-exercise hypotension (PEH) contributes to syncope which can lead to falls [48–52]. PEH causes post-exercise resetting of the baroreflex, changes in vasodilator mechanisms and alterations in metabolism which can contribute to syncope and falls [53, 54]. Management that helps to prevent post-exercise syncope may also help with the falls that occur with PEH [55].

Nocturnal Hypotension and Falls

Even though nocturnal hypotension (extreme dippers) associated with silent cerebrovascular disease, which can lead to falls, there is no study to date has looked into the association of nocturnal hypotension and falls [56].

Assessment of a Patient with Falls and Hypotensive Syndromes

A detailed falls history in the preceding 12 months including number of falls, any loss of consciousness and associated symptoms such as dizziness, light-headedness and injuries should be obtained. The history is often unreliable in the older adults because of poor recall and lack of witnesses [57]. Many elderly patients will only recall the fall but may not realise they fainted. In subjects with fall, one has to distinguish between balance-related falls (e.g. trips or slips) and unexplained falls (i.e. those preceded by dizziness or feeling faint or by no warning symptoms). Syncope is a condition that causes transient, self-limited loss of consciousness usually leading to a fall. The evaluation of syncope in the elderly should be focused on single disease like severe aortic stenosis, medications or symptomatic bradycardia or symptomatic orthostatic hypotension as the cause. So a careful history and physical exam along with targeted testing will help to identify the cause of syncope. In older adults, syncope may present in an atypical fashion or multiple abnormalities may be of concern; the assessment should be focused on these issues. In elderly subjects with gait and balance problems, moderate hemodynamic changes due to cardiovascular causes including hypotensive syndromes that are insufficient to cause syncope may cause falls [58].

Polypharmacy is an important risk factor for falls in the elderly. Medications with sedating or blood pressure lowering effects such as sedatives, anxiolytics, tricyclic antidepressants, neuroleptics and diuretics had been shown to increase the falls risk [59, 60]. A meta-analysis showed risk of falling is high with benzodiazepines (OR 1.57, 95% CI 1.43–1.72), neuroleptics and antipsychotics (OR1.59, 95% CI 1.37–1.83), antidepressants (OR 1.68, 95% CI 1.47–1.91) and diuretics (OR 1.07, 95% CI 1.01–1.14) [61].

Drop attacks are conditions which can lead to sudden leg weakness without dizziness or loss of consciousness could be due to vertebrobasilar insufficiency. Disorders affecting balance in the elderly are inner ear disorders, visual impairment, cerebral, cerebellar, spinal cord disorders, dementia, cerebrovascular disease and musculoskeletal disorders. A focused physical exam including functional assessment should be done. Identifying the multiple risk factors that contribute to falls are important. A comprehensive falls risk factor assessment should be performed in all older adults. Falls are due to multifactorial risk factors including extrinsic risk factors, intrinsic risk factors, behavioural risk factors or a combination of these (Table 16.2).

Musculoskeletal and neurological disorders along with physiological changes with ageing lead to gait disorders in the older adults. Over the age of 70 years, 35% of older adults have gait disorders [62]. With ageing, sarcopenia is seen with decrease in muscle mass and strength, decrease in visual acuity, depth perception, contrast sensitivity, decrease hearing and vestibular and somato-sensory function which can lead to gait and balance problems in older adults [63]. In some normal older adults, gait pattern consist of broad base, decrease stride length with small steps, diminish in arm swing, stooped posture with some flexion at the hips and knees, and some stiffness on turning and difficulty in performing tandem gait, which has been defined as senile or cautious gait [64, 65]. Senile gait could be an indicator of subclinical disease in older adults [66]. The abnormal gait disorders seen in older adults include antalgic gait, Trendelenburg gait, spastic gait, ataxic gait, extrapyramidal gait, high steppage gait and frontal gait [67, 68]. The features seen with different types of gait are discussed as follows:

- With extrapyramidal gait, freezing or difficulty in initiation of gait, short-stepped, shuffling, hips, knees and spine flexed, reduced arm swing, festination, en bloc turns and postural instability.

Table 16.2 Approach to the risk factor assessment of falls

(a) Intrinsic Factors
1. CNS causes: Seizures, TIA, stroke, seizures, NPH, peripheral neuropathy, cerebellar disease, parkinsonism disease
2. Decreased vision: due to cataract, glaucoma, macular degeneration and poor visual acuity
3. Inner ear causes: vertigo
4. CV causes: Aortic stenosis, arrhythmias and hypotensive syndromes
5. Abdominal causes: Incontinence
6. Musculoskeletal causes: Osteoarthritis, osteoporosis with kyphoscoliosis and foot deformities
7. Medications
(b) Extrinsic factors
1. Inappropriate foot wear
2. Rugs, slippery surfaces, poor lighting
(c) Behaviour-related risk factors
1. Hurrying or impulsivity
2. Risk taking
3. Physical inactivity
4. Fear of falling

- With antalgic gait, limping, a limited range of motion, slow and short steps, unable to bear full weight are seen.
- With ataxic gait, staggering, unsteady, falling to one side and wide-based steps are seen.
- With frontal or apraxic gait, start and turn hesitation as well as magnetic gait is seen.
- With high steppage gait, excessive flexion of hips and knees when walking, short strides, slapping quality of gait and tripping are seen with foot drop or motor neuropathy.
- In spastic gait, unilateral extension, stiff and circumduction, the arm is held in an adducted posture and is bent and rotated inwards, the forearm is pronated and the hand and the fingers are flexed, and foot is inverted and in a plantar flexed position.

The Trendelenburg gait is caused by weakness of the hip abductors, mostly the gluteal musculature, and is characterized by trunk shift over the affected hip and is best visualized from behind the patient. In a normal gait situation, both legs bear half of the body weight. When the left leg is lifted, the right leg takes the entire weight. In the Trendelenberg, it is difficult to support the body's weight on the affected side [69].

The functional tests used to do as part of the falls assessment are shown in Table 16.3.

1. Timed-Up and Go test (TUG test) score is based on the time taken by participants to rise from a chair with armrests, walk forward three metres at their usual pace, turn around and return to the chair [70]. A score of less than 10 seconds is considered normal, 15 seconds or more is abnormal and associated with an

Table 16.3 Commonly used functional assessment tools in falls

1. TUG - done by any healthcare providers
2. Functional reach tests- done by any healthcare providers
3. Tinetti Gait and Balance - done by physiotherapist (PT)
4. Berg Balance Test- done by PT
5. The Short FES-I: a shortened version of the falls efficacy scale-international to assess fear of falling- done by any healthcare providers
6. HOME FAST scale- done by occupational therapist (OT)

increased risk of falls and more than 20 seconds are associated with severe gait impairment [71]. This test has a sensitivity of 87% and specificity of also 87% in identifying older adults who are at risk for falls [72].

2. Functional reach test is measured by asking the participants to stand with their feet together, their left shoulder next to a metre ruler fixed on a wall with their left arm outstretched, and to lean forward as far as possible without losing their balance. Without moving his or her feet, the patient should reach as far forward as possible while still maintaining stability. The maximal difference between the initial ruler measurement at the fifth metacarpal head with the participant upright and leaning forward was recorded. The inability to reach at least 7 inches is highly predictive of falls in older persons. This is another reliable, valid and quick diagnostic test that evaluates balance and postural stability [73, 74].

3. Fear-of-falling is determined using the short 7-item Falls Efficacy Scale-International (short FES-I). A short FES-I score of 11 or more out of a maximum score of 28 has been considered fear-of-falling [75, 76].

4. Home Falls and Accidents Screening Tool (HOME FAST) is a 25-item checklist used to identify potential hazards in and around the home [77].

5. The Tinetti Gait and Balance Instrument is designed to determine an elders risk for falls and is usually assessed by a physiotherapist. The score for gait is 12 points while the score for Balance is 16 points with a total for the Tinetti scale is 28 points. Score of 19–24 indicates risk for falls and < 19 high risk for falls [78].

6. Berg Balance Scale is a 14-item scale designed to measure balance of the older adult by physiotherapist. The total score is 56, 41–56 = independent. 21–40 = walk with assistance, 0–20 = wheelchair bound [79] (Table 16.3).

Management

Treatment of these hypotensive syndromes usually involves a combination of education, avoidance of precipitating factors, non-pharmacological and pharmacological management and, occasionally, the insertion of permanent pacemakers in patients with cardioinhibition. For example PPH, can be treated with α-1-glucosidase inhibitors and OH with fludrocortisone or midodrine [80].

In addition, these patients may also need assistive devices, stopping the medication and also addressing the multiple comorbidities that may contribute to falls as

well as addressing home safety assessment concerns done by an occupational therapist [81]. Remove clutter, electrical cords, throw away rugs that may cause older
adults to trip. Arrange or remove furniture so there is plenty of room for walking.
Add grab bars inside and outside of your bathtub or shower and next to the toilet,
and use of high toilet seat and also high seat furniture may help with balance issues.
Lifeline with automatic fall alerts is also shown to be useful. There are challenges
associated with implementing all these interventions [82].

Conclusions

Falls are often due to multifactorial causes. The elderly are prone to hypotensive
syndromes. Falls are a leading cause of morbidity in older adults. Hypotensive
syndromes lead to cerebral hypoperfusion and subsequent falls. Identifying
optimum BP levels in these subjects must therefore prevent not only hypotension but also syncope and falls. Falls screening and falls prevention guidelines
suggest the identification of these hypotensive syndromes. A careful consideration should be given by healthcare professionals to these hypotensive syndromes especially when assessing recurrent or unexplained falls.

References

1. Tinetti ME. Falls. In: Cassel CK, et al., editors. Geriatric medicine. 2nd ed. New York:
   Springer; 1990. p. 528–34.
2. Gillespie LD, Robertson MC, Gillespie WJ, et al. Interventions for preventing falls in older
   people living in the community. Cochrane Database Syst Rev. 2012;12(9):CD007146.
3. Gomez F, Wu YY, Auais M, et al. A simple algorithm to predict falls in primary care
   patients aged 65 to 74 years: the international mobility in aging study. J Am Med Dir Assoc.
   2017;18:774–9.
4. Rubenstein LZ, Josephson KR. The epidemiology of falls and syncope. Clin Geriatr Med.
   2002;18:141–58.
5. Rapp K, Becker C, Cameron ID, et al. Epidemiology of falls in residential aged care: Analysis
   of more than 70,000 falls from residents of Bavarian Nursing Homes. J Am Med Dir Assoc.
   2012;13:187.e1–6.
6. Englander F, Hodson TJ, Terregrossa RA. Economic dimensions of slip and fall injuries. J
   Forensic Sci. 1996;41:733–46.
7. Florence CS, Bergen G, Atherly A, et al. Medical costs of fatal and nonfatal falls in older
   adults. J Am Geriatr Soc. 2018;66(4):693–8.
8. Cummings SR, Nevitt MC, Kidd S. Forgetting falls. The limited accuracy of recall of falls in
   the elderly. J Am Geriatr Soc. 1988;36:613–6.
9. Rawsky E. Review of the literature on falls among the elderly. Image J Nurs Sch.
   1998;30(1):47–52.
10. O'Loughlin J, Robitaille Y, Bovin J, Suissa S. Incidence and risk factors for falls and injurious
    falls among the community dwelling elderly. Am J Epidemiol. 1993;137:342–54.
11. Walker JE, Howland J. Falls and fear of falling among elderly persons living in the commu-
    nity: occupational therapy interventions. Am J Occup Ther. 1991;45:119–22.
12. Whipple MO, Hamel AV, Talley KMC. Fear of falling among community-dwelling older
    adults: A scoping review to identify effective evidence-based interventions. Geriatr Nurs.
    2017; https://doi.org/10.1016/j.gerinurse.2017.08.005.

13. Sakurai R, Fujiwara Y, Yasunaga M, et al. Older adults with fear of falling show deficits in motor imagery of gait. J Nutr Health Aging. 2017;21:721–6.
14. Denkinger MD, Lukas A, Nikolaus T, Hauer K. Factors associated with fear of falling and associated activity restriction in community-dwelling older adults: a systematic review. Am J Geriatr Psychiatry. 2015;23(1):72–86.
15. Hartholt KA, van Beeck EF, Polinder S, et al. Societal consequences of falls in the older population: injuries, healthcare costs, and long-term reduced quality of life. J Trauma Acute Care Surg. 2011;71(3):748–53.
16. Grafmans WC, Ooms ME, Hofstee HM, et al. Falls in the elderly: a prospective study of risk factors and risk profiles. Am J Epidemiol. 1996;143(11):1129–36.
17. Boelens C, Hekman EE, Verkerke GJ. Risk factors for falls of older citizens. Technol Health Care. 2013;21(5):521–33.
18. Raina P, Dukeshire S, Chambers L, et al. Prevalence, risk factors, and health care utilization for injuries among Canadian seniors: An analysis of 1994 National population Health Survey (IESOP Research report No. 15). Hamilton: McMaster's University; 1997.
19. Fuller GF. Falls in the elderly. Am Fam Physician. 2000;61(7):2159–68–2173-4.
20. Moncada LVV, Mire LG. Preventing falls in older persons. Am Fam Physician. 2017;96:240–7.
21. Quigley P, Bulat T, Kurtzman E, et al. Fall prevention and injury protection for nursing home residents. J Am Med Dir Assoc. 2010;11:284–93.
22. Arnold AC, Raj SR. Orthostatic hypotension: a practical approach to investigation and management. Can J Cardiol. 2017;33:1725–1728.C.
23. Zhang R, Malmstrom TK. Implications of orthostatic hypotension in older persons with and without diabetes. J Am Med Dir Assoc. 2017;18:84–5.
24. Iwanczyk L, Weintraub NT, Rubenstein LZ. Orthostatic hypotension in the nursing home setting. J Am Med Dir Assoc. 2006;7:163–7.
25. Trahair LG, Horowitz M, Jones KL. Postprandial hypotension: a systematic review. J Am Med Dir Assoc. 2014;15:394–409.
26. Pavelic A, Krbot Skoric M, Crnosija L, Habek M. Postprandial hypotension in neurological disorders; systematic review and meta-analysis. Clin Auton Res. 2017;27:263–71.
27. Lee A, Patrick P, Wishart J, et al. The effects of miglitol on glucagon-like peptide-1 secretion and appetite sensations in obese type 2 diabetics. Diabetes Obes Metab. 2002;4:329–35.
28. Willie CK, Tzeng YC, Fisher JA, et al. Integrative regulation of human brain blood flow. J Physiol. 2014;592:841–59.
29. McIntosh S, Da Costa D, Kenny RA. Outcome of an integrated approach to the investigation of dizziness, falls and syncope in elderly patients referred to a 'syncope' clinic. Age Ageing. 1993;22:53–8.
30. O'Callaghan S, Kenny RA. Neurocardiovascular instability and cognition. Yale J Biol Med. 2016;89(1):59–71.
31. Gangavati A, Hajjar I, Quach L, et al. Hypertension, orthostatic hypotension, and the risk of falls in a community-dwelling elderly population: the maintenance of balance, independent living, intellect, and zest in the elderly of Boston study. J Am Geriatr Soc. 2011;59:383–9.
32. Ooi WL, Hossain M, Lipsitz LA. The association between orthostatic hypotension and recurrent falls in nursing home residents. Am J Med. 2000;108:106–11.
33. Menant JC, Wong AK, Trollor JN, et al. Depressive symptoms and orthostatic hypotension are risk factors for unexplained falls in community-living older people. J Am Geriatr Soc. 2016;64:1073.
34. Jansen S, Bhangu J, de Rooij S, et al. The Association of Cardiovascular Disorders and Falls: a systematic review. J Am Med Dir Assoc. 2016;17:193–9.
35. Finucane C, O'Connell M, Donoghue O, et al. Impaired orthostatic blood pressure recovery is associated with unexplained and injurious falls. J Am Geriatr Soc. 2017;65:474–82.
36. Consensus statement on the definition of orthostatic hypotension, pure autonomic failure, and multiple system atrophy. The Consensus Committee of the American Autonomic Society and the American Academy of Neurology. Neurology. 1996;46:1470.

37. Freeman R, Wieling W, Axelrod FB, et al. Consensus statement on the definition of orthostatic hypotension, neutrally mediated syncope and the postural tachycardia syndrome. Clin Auton Res. 2011;21:69–72.
38. McDonald D, Pearce M, Kerr SR, Newton J. A prospective study of the association between orthostatic hypotension and falls: definition matters. Age Ageing. 2016;46(3):439–45.
39. Hartog LC, Schrijnders D, Landman GWD. Is orthostatic hypotension related to falling? A meta-analysis of individual patient data of prospective observational studies. Age Ageing. 2017;46:568–75.
40. Yatsuya H, Folsom AR, Alonso A, et al. Postural changes in blood pressure and incidence of ischemic stroke subtypes: the ARIC Study. Hypertension. 2011;57:167–73.
41. Callisaya ML, Beare R, Phan T, et al. Progression of white matter hyperintensities of presumed vascular origin increases the risk of falls in older people. J Gerontol A Biol Sci Med Sci. 2015;70:360–6.
42. Masuo K, Mikami H, Ogihara T, et al. Changes in frequency of orthostatic hypotension in elderly hypertensive patients under medications. Am J Hypertens. 1996;9:263–8.
43. Jonsson PV, Lipsitz LA, Kelley M, Koestner J. Hypotensive responses to common daily activities in institutionalized elderly. A potential risk for recurrent falls. Arch Intern Med. 1990;150:1518–24.
44. Jansen RW, Connelly CM, Kelley-Gagnon MM, et al. Postprandial hypotension in elderly patients with unexplained syncope. Arch Intern Med. 1995;155:945–52.
45. Aronow WS, Ahn C. Postprandial hypotension in 499 elderly persons in a long-term health care facility. J Am Geriatr Soc. 1994;42:930–2.
46. Le Couteur DG, Fisher AA, Davis MW, McLean AJ. Postprandial systolic blood pressure responses of older people in residential care: association with risk of falling. Gerontology. 2003;49:260–4.
47. Tan MP, Newton JL, Chadwick TJ, Parry SW. The relationship between carotid sinus hypersensitivity, orthostatic hypotension, and vasovagal syncope: a case–control study. Europace. 2008;10(12):1400–5.
48. Anunciação PG, Polito MD. A review on post-exercise hypotension in hypertensive individuals. Arq Bras Cardiol. 2011;96:425–6.
49. Kenny MJ, Seals DR. Postexercise hypotension: key features, mechanisms, and clinical significance. Hypertension. 1993;22:653–64.
50. MacDonald JR. Potential causes, mechanisms, and implications of post exercise hypotension. J Hum Hypertens. 2002;16:225–36.
51. Krediet CTP, Wilde AAM, Halliwill JR, Wieling W. Syncope during exercise, documented with continuous blood pressure monitoring during ergometer testing. Clin Auton Res. 2005;15:59–62.
52. Krediet CTP, Wilde AAM, Wieling W, Halliwill JR. Exercise related syncope, when it's not the heart. Clin Auton Res. 2004;14(1):25–36.
53. Mündel T, Perry BG, Ainslie PN, et al. Post exercise orthostatic intolerance: influence of exercise intensity. Exp Physiol. 2015;100(8):915–25.
54. de Brito LC, Rezende RA, da Silva Junior ND, et al. Post-exercise hypotension and its mechanisms differ after morning and evening exercise: a randomized crossover study. PLoS One. 2015;10(7):e0132458.
55. O'Connor FG, Levine BD, Childress MA, et al. Practical management: a systematic approach to the evaluation of exercise-related syncope in athletes. Clin J Sport Med. 2009;19:429–34.
56. Kario K, Matsuo T, Kobayashi H, et al. Nocturnal fall of blood pressure and silent cerebrovascular damage in elderly hypertensive patients. Advanced silent cerebrovascular damage in extreme dippers. Hypertension. 1996;27(1):130–5.
57. O'Dwyer C, Bennett K, Langan Y, et al. Amnesia for loss of consciousness is common in vasovagal syncope. Europace. 2011;13:1040–5.
58. Kenny RA, Parry SW. Syncope-related falls in the elderly. J Geriatr Cardiol. 2005;2:74–83.

59. Richardson K, Bennett K, Kenny RA. Polypharmacy including falls risk-increasing medications and subsequent falls in community-dwelling middle-aged and older adults. Age Ageing. 2015;44(1):90–6.
60. Park H, Satoh H, Miki A, et al. Medications associated with falls in older people: systematic review of publications from a recent 5 year period. Eur J Clin Pharmacol. 2015;71(12):1429–40.
61. Woolcott JC, Richardson KJ, Wiens MO, et al. Meta-analysis of the impact of 9 medications classes on falls in elderly patients. Arch Intern Med. 2009;169:1952–60.
62. Verghese J, Levalley A, Hall CB, et al. Epidemiology of gait disorders in community residing older adults. J Am Geriatr Soc. 2006;54(2):255–61.
63. Judge JO, Ounuu S, Davis RB. Effects of age in the biomechanics and physiology of gait. Clin Geriatr Med. 1996;12(4):659–78.
64. Eible RJ, Hughes L, Higgins C. The syndrome of senile gait. J Neurol. 1992;239:71–5.
65. Hageman PA. Gait characteristics in healthy elderly; a literature review. Section of geriatrics. Am Physiol Therapy Assoc. 1995;18:2–5.
66. Bloem BR, Gussekloo J, Lagaay AM, et al. Idiopathic senile gait disorders are signs of subclinical disease. J Am Geriatr Soc. 2000;48(9):1098–101.
67. Num JC, Marsden CD, Thompson PD. Human walking and higher- level gait disorders particularly in the elderly. Neurology. 1993;43(2):268–79.
68. Alexander NB. Gait disorders in older adults. J Am Geriatr Soc. 1996;44(4):434–51.
69. Lim MR, Huang RC, Wu A, et al. Evaluation of the elderly patient with an abnormal gait. J Am Acad Orthop Surg. 2007;15(2):107–17.
70. Schoene D, Wu SM, Mikolaizak AS, et al. Discriminative ability and predictive validity of the timed up and go test in identifying older people who fall: systematic review and meta-analysis. J Am Geriatr Soc. 2013;61(2):202–8.
71. Podsiadlo D, Richardson S. The timed "Up & Go": a test of basic functional mobility for frail elderly persons. J Am Geriatr Soc. 1991;39(2):142–8.
72. Shumway-Cook A, Brauer S, Woollacott M. Predicting the probability for falls in community-dwelling older adults using the Timed Up & Go Test. Phys Ther. 2000;80(9):896–903.
73. Perell KL, Nelson A, Goldman RL, et al. Fall risk assessment measures: an analytic review. J Gerontol A Biol Sci Med Sci. 2001;56(12):M761–6.
74. Duncan PW, Weiner DK, Chandler J, Studenski S. Functional reach: a new clinical measure of balance. J Gerontol. 1990;45(6):M192–7.
75. Delbaere K, Close JCT, Mikolaizak AS, et al. The Falls Efficacy Scale International (FES-I). A comprehensive longitudinal validation study. Age Ageing. 2010;14(2):210–6.
76. Hauer KA, Kempen GIJM, Schwenk M, et al. Validity and sensitivity to change of the falls efficacy scales international to assess fear of falling in older adults with and without cognitive impairment. Gerontology. 2011;14(5):462–72.
77. Mackenzie L, Byles J, Higginbotham N. Reliability of the Home Falls and Accidents Screening Tool (HOME FAST) for identifying older people at increased risk of falls. Disabil Rehabil. 2002;24(5):266–74.
78. Tinetti ME, Williams TF, Mayewski R. Fall risk index for elderly patients based on number of chronic disabilities. Am J Med. 1986;80:429–34.
79. Berg K, Wood-Dauphinee S, Williams JI, Maki B. Measuring balance in the elderly: validation of an instrument. Can. J Pub Health. 1992;2:S7–11.
80. Alagiakrishnan K. Current pharmacological management of hypotensive syndromes in the elderly. Drugs Aging. 2015;32(5):337–48.
81. Campbell AJ, Robertson MC. Rethinking individual and community fall prevention strategies: a meta-regression comparing single and multifactorial interventions. Age Ageing. 2007;36(6):656–62.
82. Moore M, Williams B, Ragsdale S, et al. Translating a multifactorial fall prevention intervention into practice: a controlled evaluation of a fall prevention clinic. J Am Geriatr Soc. 2010;58(2):357–63.

Hypotensive Syndromes and Cognitive Impairment/Dementia

Kannayiram Alagiakrishnan and Kamal Masaki

Introduction

Both hypertension and hypotension have been associated with dementia, and blood pressure can be a double-edged sword with the risk of contributing to cognitive decline. Dementia is a major health problem throughout the world and also the leading cause of disability in the elderly. It causes global deterioration of cognition and makes one dependent for day-to-day functioning. The prevalence of dementia doubles every 5 years in persons aged 65–90 years [1]. By 2050, 1 in 85 persons worldwide will be living with Alzheimer disease [2]. Different hypotensive syndromes can affect the brain depending on the magnitude, frequency, and duration of these conditions individually and together. The duration of hypotensive episodes due to these conditions last from a few seconds with carotid sinus syndrome (CSS) to minutes with orthostatic hypotension (OH) and postprandial hypotension (PPH). In addition, these hypotensive conditions can occur alone or in combination. In this chapter, the authors discuss the role of different hypotensive syndromes in cognitive decline and dementia.

Orthostatic Hypotension and Cognitive Impairment/ Dementia

According to a study by Viramo et al., prevalence of OH increased steeply with age among individuals in the community. This study showed no overall association between OH and cognitive decline after two years [3]. In the Rotterdam study, having orthostatic hypotension at the start of the study increased the risk of developing

K. Alagiakrishnan (✉)
Division of Geriatric Medicine, University of Alberta, Edmonton, AB, Canada

K. Masaki
Division of Geriatric Medicine, University of Hawaii at Manoa, Honolulu, HI, USA

© Springer Nature Switzerland AG 2020
K. Alagiakrishnan, M. Banach (eds.), *Hypotensive Syndromes in Geriatric Patients*, https://doi.org/10.1007/978-3-030-30332-7_17

dementia over the next 25 years by 15%, with similar results for all-cause dementia and Alzheimer disease. In this study, OH was found to be associated with long-term risk of dementia, independent of various other risk factors. Greater risk of dementia was seen with greater orthostatic drop of SBP ($p = 0.02$), as well as among those who lacked a compensatory increase in heart rate ($p = 0.05$) [4]. Other studies found that OH increased the risk of conversion from mild cognitive impairment to dementia after 3 years [5] and also increased risk of dementia in patients with Parkinson disease [6]. Only one other study has assessed the longitudinal relationship between OH and the risk of dementia in initially healthy individuals. In a sample of 1480 individuals in the Swedish general population, OH was associated with an increased risk of having dementia at re-examination after 6 years. In this study, subclinical OH (defined as a systolic BP drop <20 mmHg or diastolic BP drop <10 mm Hg but with symptoms like dizziness, fatigue, and light-headedness) was also associated with significantly increased risk of MCI [7]. However, the investigators were unable to fit survival models or adjust for cardiovascular risk factors aside from hypertension, and attrition was substantial, with 37.5% of participants lost to follow-up [7]. One study by Tanaka et al. in patients with Parkinson disease suggested a relationship between a riser pattern (nighttime blood pressure higher than daytime blood pressure) and dementia, particularly in those with coexisting orthostatic hypotension ($p < 0.01$) [8]. In a cross-sectional study by Frewen et al. on 4690 subjects, OH coupled with supine HTN was associated with lower cognitive performance [9]. Yap et al. in their longitudinal study over 1–2 years showed hypotension with OH significantly increased the risk of cognitive impairment compared to subjects with hypertension and OH [10]. In the Maine-Syracuse Longitudinal Study, systolic orthostatic hypotension was significantly associated with reduced cognitive function [11].

A few studies have investigated OH in relation to cognitive test performance. In the ARIC study, OH was associated with decline in two cognitive tests, but this decline was largely explained by cardiovascular risk factors [12]. In another study, orthostatic hypotension was associated with executive dysfunction in mild cognitive impairment [13]. In the Progetto Veneto Anziani study, OH was associated with cognitive decline (CD; defined as a drop of ≥ 3 points in the MMSE from baseline to follow-up over 4.4 ± 1.2 years), but not with cognitive impairment (CI; adjusted MMSE score ≤ 24) [14]. In the DANTE (Discontinuation of Antihypertensive Treatment in Elderly people) RCT study, recovery from orthostatic hypotension was significantly higher in persons who completely discontinued all antihypertensive medication (61%) compared with the continuation group (38%) [RR = 1.60 (95% CI = 1.10–2.31); $P = 0.01$] among those with mild cognitive impairment [15]. In a recent study using this cohort, OH was not associated with decreased cognitive functioning or decreased cerebral blood flow and ischemic brain damage. The study limitations were that it was a cross-sectional study, and all older subjects were using antihypertensive medications [16]. A cross-sectional study by Frewen et al. showed that OH was associated with worse global cognitive function and memory independent of potential confounders in women [17].

The Irish Longitudinal Study showed no association between impaired recovery of orthostatic BP and change in cognition over a two-year period [18]. The recent community-based Three-City Study elderly cohort showed that OH at baseline increased the risk of developing dementia over 12 years by 25% ($p = 0.04$) [19]. Studies on OH and cognitive impairment and dementia are summarized in Table 17.1.

Table 17.1 Studies on OH and CI/dementia

Name of the study	Type	Sample size	Age in years	Follow-up	Outcomes
Frewen et al. (2014) [9]	Cross-sectional	1868	62.8 ± 8.7	–	OH with supine hypertension was associated with decreased global cognitive function, Beta = −0.15, 99% CI = −0.29, −0.14, $p = 0.004$ Decreased executive function, Beta = 0.11, 99% CI = 0.22–0.11, $p = 0.006$
Bocti et al. (2017) [13]	Cross-sectional	120	75.5 ± 9.2	–	In MCI subjects, OH was associated with lower cognitive performance Visual working memory ($p < 0.001$), processing speed ($p = 0.006$), stroop flexibility ($p = 0.030$), trail-making test part B ($p = 0.024$)
Dante study (2018) [15]	Cross-sectional	420	Mean age 81	–	OH was not associated with decreased cognitive function
Viramo et al. (1999) [3]	Prospective cohort	1159	76 ± 4.9	2 years	OH did not predict cognitive decline
Yap et al. (2008) [10]	Prospective cohort	2321	Mean age 65.5	1–2 years	OH with hypotension increased the risk of cognitive impairment, OR = 4.1, 95% CI = 1.11–15.1.
ARIC study (2010) [12]	Prospective cohort	10,572	45–64	6 years	OH was not associated with Delayed recall, OR = 1.08, 95% CI = 0.86–1.35 Digital symbol substitution, OR = 1.05, 95% CI = 0.83–1.35 Word fluency, OR = 1.03, 95% CI = 0.80–1.31

(continued)

Table 17.1 (continued)

Name of the study	Type	Sample size	Age in years	Follow-up	Outcomes
Anang JBM et al. (2014) [6]	Prospective cohort	80	70.5 ± 7.02	4.4 years	Increased dementia risk in PD subjects, OR = 4.80, 95% CI = 2.00–11.40, $p = 0.003$
Good aging in Skane study (GAS-SNAC) (2014) [7]	Prospective cohort	1480	60–93	6 years	MCI risk with subclinical OH, OR = 1.84, 95% CI = 1.20–2.80 Dementia risk with OH, OR = 1.93, 95% CI = 1.19– 3.14
Hayakawa et al. (2015) [5]	Case-control study	Case (MCI)- 150, control −75	74 ± 6.8	3 years	MCI conversion to dementia HR = 2.77, 95% CI = 1.02–7.50
Progetto Veneto Anziani (PRO VA) study (2016) [14]	Prospective cohort	1408	71.4 ± 5.0	4.4 years	OH with cognitive impairment, OR = 0.99, 95% CI = 0.85–1.15, $p = 0.86$. OH with cognitive decline, OR = 1.50, 95% CI = 1.26–1.78, $p < 0.0001$
Rotterdam study (2016) [4]	Prospective cohort	6204	68.5± 8.6	25 years	OH at baseline increased risk for dementia HR = 1.15, 95% CI = 1.00– 1.34, $p = 0.05$
The Irish-longitudinal study on ageing (2016) [18]	Prospective Cohort	4894	65.4 ± 9.1	2 years	No association between impaired recovery of orthostatic BP and change in cognition
Three city study (2017) [19]	Prospective cohort	7425	65 and above	12 years	OH at baseline increased risk of dementia HR = 1.24, 95% CI = 1.02– 1.52, $p = 0.04$

Mechanisms of OH Causing Cognitive Decline

Orthostatic hypotension is a common cause of transient cerebral hypoperfusion that is associated with subclinical brain injury, as well as increased risk of stroke, and recurrent episodes can cause brain damage. Autonomic nervous system function is responsible for maintaining continuous cerebral perfusion, together with local vasoreactivity, which has previously been associated with increased risk of dementia in the general population [20]. Brief episodes of hypoperfusion elicited by sudden blood pressure drops may lead to hypoxia, with detrimental effects on brain tissue through ischemia, neuroinflammation, and oxidative stress [21]. These mechanisms have been suggested to be of particular relevance in the pathogenesis of small vessel disease [22] and orthostatic blood pressure drops in patients with dementia have been associated with presence of deep white matter and basal ganglia hyperintensities [23], but not with volume of white matter hyperintensities [24]. The reduction in cerebral blood flow with autonomic failure has also been reported to predominantly affect the hippocampus [25], possibly linking hypoperfusion to early Alzheimer pathology. OH serves as a marker of other detrimental consequences of autonomic dysfunction, such as blood pressure variability [26, 27], response to Valsalva manoeuvre [28, 29], cardiovascular reflex, and heart rate variability [30, 31]. There could be other pathways linked to dementia other than hypoperfusion. For example, decreased arterial wall compliance with hypertension likely contributes to OH by diminishing baroreceptor sensitivity [32]. Arterial wall stiffness and OH are both associated with increased burden of cerebral white matter lesions (WMLs) and vascular disease including stroke [33–36]. Autoregulation of brain circulation allows maintenance of constant cerebral blood flow over a wide range of blood pressures (approximately 80 to 200 mmHg). Alzheimer's Disease causes acetylcholine deficits and acetylcholine has been shown to regulate cerebral blood flow through parasympathetic innervation and causes arterial relaxation by promoting the synthesis of vasodilator agents. The autodysregulation and acetylcholine deficits may contribute to hypotension [37]. The prevalence of hypotension, including OH, was shown in up to 50% of subjects with vascular dementia [38]. A lack of symptoms with orthostasis was previously observed in patients with dementia [39] and may warrant caution in view of studies linking low blood pressure in late life to cognitive decline and dementia [40]. OH most commonly arises due to autonomic dysfunction in the absence of neurological disease, but may be provoked by synucleinopathies (e.g., Parkinson disease), small fibre peripheral neuropathy, volume depletion (e.g., due to diuretics), and diminished cardiac pump function. In addition, several drugs can cause or aggravate OH, including antihypertensive agents and antidepressants. Participants in one study with heart failure at baseline seemed particularly affected by OH, possibly due to the lack of a compensatory increase in stroke volume. OH has been associated with the development of structural cardiac changes, including left ventricular hypertrophy [41], which may function as a mediator towards dementia [42, 43].

In Andin et al.'s retrospective study, he examined various cardiovascular risk factors and correlated them with WMD and Alzheimer disease findings. The prevalence of HTN ($p = 0.006$), OH ($p = 0.024$), and dizziness/unsteadiness ($p = 0.001$) was more common in people with both WMD and AD compared to those with just AD without WMD [44]. In Raiha et al.'s retrospective study, they read CT scans and clinical charts of 251 older subjects. WMLs were more common in people with vascular (69.8%) and mixed dementia (69.2%). WMLs were more common in people with heart failure ($p = 0.0012$) and OH ($p = 0.036$). In addition, systolic

($p = 0.0069$) and diastolic ($p = 0.031$) values of low blood pressure were both associated with WML. Hypoperfusion of the brain may be the cause of WMLs [45]. Kario et al. did MRI scans on senior patients with sustained hypertension and found that WMLs and silent cerebral infarcts were more common in people with orthostatic hypotension ($p = 0.04$) or orthostatic hypertension ($p < 0.0001$) than in people without these syndromes [46]. In Matsubayashi et al.'s retrospective study, he divided healthy community-living seniors into three groups: normal blood pressure, postural hypotension, and postural hypertension. People with normal blood pressure scored better on the Hasegawa Dementia Scale ($p = 0.0333$) and computer-assisted visuospatial cognitive performance test ($p = 0.0001$) compared to the other two groups. People with postural hypotension or postural hypertension had more severe WMLs ($p = 0.001$) [47].

OH was also related to arterial stiffness in older adults [48]. In a small study, Augmentation Index (AI) and Pulse Pressure Amplification (PPA), which are markers of vascular stiffness, were associated with poor executive function and language cognitive domain deficits [49]. Meta-analyses have also shown that arterial stiffness can contribute to cognitive decline and dementia [50, 51].

Postprandial Hypotension and Dementia

Idiaquez, Rios, and Sandoval (1997) found postprandial hypotension in patients with Alzheimer disease, with a fall in blood pressure of 20 mmHg or more after meals. Maximum blood pressure fall in AD patients was observed between 20 and 120 minutes after food ingestion. The authors suggested that postprandial hypotension in AD may be due to abnormalities in cardiac vasomotor regulation, gut peptide liberation, or both [52]. Idiaquez et al. (2007) reported no consistent association between OH or PPH and cognitive deficits in Parkinson disease [53].

In patients with dementia with Lewy bodies (DLB), postprandial and orthostatic hypotension contributes to cognitive decline. However, these aspects of the condition might be treatable. A case report of postprandial hypotension and orthostatic hypotension due to autonomic dysfunction in a patient with dementia with Lewy bodies found that the administration of the DPP-4 inhibitor sitagliptin improved the patient's postprandial hypotensive episodes, as well as her episodes of orthostatic hypotension, by modifying the reactivity of her sympathetic nervous system. The patient did not suffer any adverse effects of sitagliptin treatment. The amelioration of the patient's hypotensive episodes led to an improvement in her cognitive function [54].

Carotid Sinus Hypersensitivity and Dementia

Carotid sinus hypersensitivity (CSH) has been associated with DLB, Parkinson dementia, and AD. In one study, CSH was seen in 11.1% of AD and 32% of DLB when compared to 3.2% of controls [55]. Degeneration of the medullary autonomic nuclei may be responsible for the pathogenesis of CSH. Symptoms include retrograde amnesia with loss of consciousness and unexplained falls with cognitive impairment [56].

Kenny et al. found the severity of WMD on MRI correlated with systolic blood pressure drops during carotid sinus stimulation (R = 0.58, p < 0.005) in dementia secondary to neurocardiovascular disability. There may be a link between bradycardia-induced hypotension and WMD, and the possibility of neurocardiovascular instability leads to cognitive impairment and dementia. Perhaps interventions that prevent a drop in heart rate would benefit cognitive function [57]. Ballard et al. did a retrospective study on dementia subjects and found that systolic blood pressure (BP) drop >30 mm Hg during carotid sinus massage was associated with basal ganglia (OR = 11.0, 95% CI = 1.2–99.5) and deep white matter (OR = 10.0, 95% CI = 1.8–55.7) MRI hyperintensities [58].

Combined Hypotensive Syndromes and Dementia

Schoon et al. performed a study in 184 subjects, of which 73 subjects had 2 hypotensive syndromes (OH and PPH in 34, OH and CSH in 23, and PPH and CSH in 16) and 27 patients had all 3 hypotensive syndromes. The prevalence of cognitive impairment did not differ among patients with none, one, two, or three hypotensive syndromes. During testing, hypotensive symptoms were reported by 40% of patients with OH, 62% of patients with PPH, and 14% of patients with CSH. Cognitive impairment/dementia did not influence the report of hypotensive symptoms. The limitation of this study is that it is a retrospective study with a cross-sectional design and small numbers in each group. MMSE was used to assess cognitive function, and this test has its own limitations [59].

Hypotension Due to Vasovagal Syncope and Dementia

Vasovagal syncope is a common cause of fainting in individuals. In the TILDA study, in individuals above the age of 50 years, syncope and unexplained falls were independently associated with worse cognitive performance [60].

Post-Exercise Hypotension and Dementia

Recovery from exercise refers to the time period between the end of a bout of exercise and the subsequent return to a resting or recovered state. Hemodynamic adjustments and the underlying causes that drive cardiovascular recovery highlight how they differ following resistance and aerobic exercise. The hypotensive effects of aerobic and resistance exercise and associated mechanisms, if left unchecked, can progress to symptomatic hypotension and syncope [61].

There is evidence that exercise reduces cognitive decline in healthy older adults [62] and those with mild cognitive impairment [63] and that aerobic exercise can alter brain structure and function [64]. Even though exercise has been shown to improve cognition, no studies have looked at the effects of post-exercise hypotension on cognition.

Nocturnal Hypotension and Dementia

In the J-SHIPP study, abnormal nocturnal BP profile, including extreme dippers, was found to be a strong indicator of MCI in otherwise apparently healthy community-dwelling elderly persons [65].

Limitations of the Studies

Missed diagnosis of hypotensive syndromes may result in misclassification, and missed diagnosis of cognitive dysfunction or decline may contribute to the underestimation of the true association or effect. The impact of a hypotensive episode on the brain depends on its magnitude and duration. With cross-sectional study design, the duration of hypotensive syndromes is unknown. Most studies have not used standardized criteria to diagnose MCI and dementia in these hypotensive syndrome subjects. Some studies have adjusted for vascular and other risk factors that contribute to cognitive decline, but residual confounding might have occurred because of the lack of adjustment for all confounding factors that may contribute to cognitive decline. Moreover, mood and functional evaluations have not been done in these studies, which can confound the assessment of CI.

Recommended Cognitive Testing in Patients with Hypotensive Syndromes

Cognitive decline in hypotensive syndromes can affect different domains of cognition like memory, attention, learning, motor speed, reaction time, and executive functioning. Healthcare professionals should become familiar with cognitive tests to screen for MCI and dementia. The common clinical cognitive screening tests used in primary care clinical practice are the Mini-Cog [66], the Mini-Mental State Examination (MMSE) [67], the Montreal Cognitive Assessment (MoCA) [68], the Saint Louis University Mental Status (SLUMS) examination [69], and General Practitioner Assessment of Cognition (GPCOG) [70]. Different screening tools to detect cognitive impairment have varying levels of ease of use, efficacy, sensitivity, and specificity. The Mini-Cog is a brief cognitive screen that combines three-item recall and clock drawing [66]. The MMSE has been used as a global screening tool for cognitive impairment for over three decades, but is not sensitive enough to pick up subtle cognitive deficits [67]. The MoCA was developed to screen for MCI and measures seven cognitive domains, including domains not measured by the MMSE like executive function and abstraction [68]. Frontal Assessment Battery (FAB) is a cognitive test to assess frontal lobe, mainly executive function [71]. More extensive cognitive testing can be done using The Modified Mini-Mental State (MMMS, or 3MS) test [72], the Cognitive Abilities Screening Instrument (CASI) [73], the Cognistat [74], and the Executive Interview (EXIT) [75].

Although all these tools may give some idea about cognitive status, they are not diagnostic tests. Definitive diagnosis requires the use of standardized criteria, such as the Petersen criteria and Europe Consortium criteria for MCI, and DSM IV criteria for dementia [76–78]. Some studies for suspected cases of cognitive impairment with hypotensive syndromes have used DSM criteria for the final diagnosis of dementia, NINDS-ADRDA criteria for Alzheimer disease, and NINDS-AIREN criteria for vascular dementia [79, 80]. For staging of dementia, the Clinical Dementia Rating (CDR) scale can be used [81]. Table 17.2 lists some of the commonly used screening tools for cognitive impairment and dementia, which can be used in subjects with hypotensive syndromes.

Table 17.2 Cognitive tests that can be used in patients with hypotensive syndromes

Screening or brief assessment tools
sMMSE: Standardized mini-mental status examination
MoCA: Montreal cognitive assessment
Mini-cog
SLUMS: Saint-Louis University mental status exam
GPCOG: The general practitioner assessment of cognition
FAB: Frontal assessment battery
Extended testing of global cognitive function
3MS: The modified mini-mental state (MMMS, or 3MS) test
CASI: Cognitive abilities screening instrument
Cognistat
EXIT (executive interview)
Diagnostic criteria
European consortium Criteria or Petersen criteria for MCI
DSM IV criteria for dementia
National Institute of neurological and communicative disorders and stroke and the Alzheimer's disease and related disorders association (NINDS-ADRDA) criteria for Alzheimer's disease
NINDS-AIREN criteria for vascular dementia
Staging of dementia
CDR (clinical Dementia rating) scale

Conclusion

While the results of the studies are mixed, evidence from several longitudinal cohort studies shows that OH in the elderly increases the risk of developing cognitive decline and dementia. OH measurements could help to identify elderly subjects at higher risk of developing dementia. Understanding of the association between hypotensive syndromes and cognitive impairment and dementia will improve overall management. Caution should be used with excessive BP lowering with antihypertensive medications in older patients. Optimal control of blood pressure should be exploited for its potential to reduce future cognitive impairment. The effect of treatment of orthostatic hypotension on markers of neurodegenerative disease and cognition needs to be further investigated. In patients with hypotension-related syncope and dementia, there should be careful consideration before initiating cholinesterase inhibitors for the treatment of dementia.

References

1. Jorm AF, Jolley D. The incidence of dementia: a meta-analysis. Neurology. 1998;51:728–33.
2. Brookmeyer R, Johnson E, Ziegler-Graham K, et al. Forecasting the global burden of Alzheimer's disease. Alzheimer's & Dementia. J Alzheimer's Assoc. 2007;3(1):186–91.
3. Viramo P, Luukinen H, Koski K, Laippala P, Sulkava R, Kivelä SL. Orthostatic hypotension and cognitive decline in older people. J Am Geriatr Soc. 1999;47:600–4.
4. Wolters FJ, Mattace-Raso FUS, Koudstaal PJ, Hofman A, Ikram MA. Heart brain connection collaborative research group orthostatic hypotension and the long-term risk of dementia: a population-based study. PLoS Med. 2016;13(10):e1002143.
5. Hayakawa T, McGarrigle CA, Coen RF, Soraghan CJ, Foran T, Lawlor BA, et al. Orthostatic blood pressure behavior in people with mild cognitive impairment predicts conversion to dementia. J Am Geriatr Soc. 2015;63:1868–73.
6. Anang JBM, Gagnon J-F, Bertrand J-A, Romenets SR, Latreille V, Panisset M, et al. Predictors of dementia in Parkinson disease: a prospective cohort study. Neurology. 2014 Sep 30;83:1253–60.
7. Elmståhl S, Widerström E. Orthostatic intolerance predicts mild cognitive impairment: incidence of mild cognitive impairment and dementia from the Swedish general population cohort good aging in Skåne. Clin Interv Aging. 2014;9:1993–2002.
8. Tanaka R, Shimo Y, Yamashiro K, Ogawa T, Nishioka K, Oyama G, Umemura A, Hattori N. Association between abnormal nocturnal blood pressure profile and dementia in Parkinson's disease. Parkinsonism and Related Disorders. 2018;46:24–9.
9. Frewen J, Finucane C, Savva GM, Boyle G, Kenny RA. Orthostatic hypotension is associated with lower cognitive performance in adults aged 50 plus with supine hypertension. J Gerontol A Biol Sci Med Sci. 2014;69(7):878–85.
10. Yap PLK, Niti M, Yap KB, Ng TP. Orthostatic hypotension, hypotension and cognitive status: early comorbid markers of primary dementia? Dement Geriatr Cogn Disord. 2008;26:239–46.
11. Torres RV, Elias MF, Crichton GE, Dore GA, Davey A. Systolic orthostatic hypotension is related to lowered cognitive function: findings from the Maine-Syracuse longitudinal study. J Clin Hypertens. 2017 Dec;19(12):1357–65.
12. Rose KM, Couper D, Eigenbrodt ML, Mosley TH, Sharrett AR, Gottesman RF. Orthostatic hypotension and cognitive function: the atherosclerosis risk in communities study. Neuroepidemiology. 2010;34:1–7.

13. Bocti C, Pépin F, Tétreault M, Cossette P, Langlois F, Imbeault H, Duval N, Lacombe G, Fulop TJ. Orthostatic hypotension associated with executive dysfunction in mild cognitive impairment. Neurol Sci. 2017 Nov 15;382:79–83.
14. Curreri C, Giantin V, Veronese N, et al. Orthostatic changes in blood pressure and cognitive status in the elderly. The Progetto Veneto Anziani study. Hypertension. 2016;68:427–35.
15. Mooneni JEF, Foster- Dingley JC, Ruijter WD, et al. Effect of discontinuation of antihypertensive medication on orthostatic hypotension in older persons with mild cognitive impairment: the DANTE study Leiden. Age Ageing. 2016;45:249–55.
16. Foster- Dingley JC, Moonen JEF, DeRuijter W, et al. Orthostatic hypotension in older persons is not associated with cognitive functioning features of cerebral damage or cerebral blood flow. J Hypertens. 2018;36:1201–6.
17. Frewen J, Savva GM, Boyle G, Finucane C, Kenny RA. Cognitive performance in orthostatic hypotension: findings from a nationally representative sample. J Am Geriatr Soc. 2014;62(1):117–22.
18. Feeney J, O'Leary N, Kenny RA. Impaired orthostatic blood pressure recovery and cognitive performance at two- year follow- up in older adults: the Irish longitudinal study on ageing. Clin Auton Res. 2016;26:127–33.
19. Cremer A, Sounare A, Berr C, et al. Orthostatic hypotension and risk of incident dementia- results from a 12- year follow- up of the Three-City study cohort. Hypertension. 2017;70(1):44–9.
20. Wolters FJ, De Bruijn RF, Hofman A, Koudstaal PJ, Ikram MA. Heart brain connection collaborative research group. Cerebral vasoreactivity, apolipoprotein E, and the risk of dementia: a population-based study. Arterioscler Thromb Vasc Biol. 2016;36:204–10.
21. Raz L, Knoefel J, Bhaskar K. The neuropathology and cerebrovascular mechanisms of dementia. J Cereb Blood Flow Metab. 2016;36:172–86.
22. Wardlaw JM, Smith C, Dichgans M. Mechanisms of sporadic cerebral small vessel disease: insights from neuroimaging. Lancet Neurol. 2013;12:483–97.
23. Ballard C, O'Brien J, Barber B, Scheltens P, Shaw F, McKeith I, et al. Neurocardiovascular instability, hypotensive episodes, and MRI lesions in neurodegenerative dementia. Ann N Y Acad Sci. 2000;903:442–5.
24. Soennesyn H, Nilsen DW, Oppedal K, Greve OJ, Beyer MK, Aarsland D. Relationship between orthostatic hypotension and white matter hyperintensity load in older patients with mild dementia. PLoS One. 2012;7:e52196.
25. Laosiripisan J, Tarumi T, Gonzales MM, Haley AP, Tanaka H. Association between cardiovagal baroreflex sensitivity and baseline cerebral perfusion of the hippocampus. Clin Auton Res. 2015;25:213–8.
26. Alpérovitch A, Blachier M, Soumaré A, Ritchie K, Dartigues J-F, Richard-Harston S, et al. Blood pressure variability and risk of dementia in an elderly cohort, the Three-City study. Alzheimers Dement. 2014;10(5 Suppl):S330–7.
27. Yamaguchi Y, Wada M, Sato H, Nagasawa H, Koyama S, Takahashi Y, et al. Impact of ambulatory blood pressure variability on cerebral small vessel disease progression and cognitive decline in community-based elderly Japanese. Am J Hypertens. 2014;27:1257–67.
28. Jensen-Dahm C, Waldemar G, Staehelin Jensen T, Malmqvist L, Moeller MM, Andersen BB, et al. Autonomic dysfunction in patients with mild to moderate Alzheimer's disease. J Alzheimers Dis. 2015;47:681–9.
29. Algotsson A, Viitanen M, Winblad B, Solders G. Autonomic dysfunction in Alzheimer's disease. Acta Neurol Scand. 1995;91:14–8.
30. Collins O, Dillon S, Finucane C, Lawlor B, Kenny RA. Parasympathetic autonomic dysfunction is common in mild cognitive impairment. Neurobiol Aging. 2012;33:2324–33.
31. Idiaquez J, Sandoval E, Seguel A. Association between neuropsychiatric and autonomic dysfunction in Alzheimer's disease. Clin Auton Res. 2002;12:43–6.
32. Mattace-Raso FU, Van den Meiracker AH, Bos WJ, Van der Cammen TJ, Westerhof BE, Elias-Smale S, et al. Arterial stiffness, cardiovagal baroreflex sensitivity and postural blood pressure changes in older adults: the Rotterdam study. J Hypertens. 2007;25:1421–6.

33. Angelousi A, Girerd N, Benetos A, Frimat L, Gautier S, Weryha G, et al. Association between orthostatic hypotension and cardiovascular risk, cerebrovascular risk, cognitive decline and falls as well as overall mortality: a systematic review and meta-analysis. J Hypertens. 2014;32:1562–71.
34. Ballard C, O'Brien J, Barber B, Scheltens P, Shaw F, McKeith I, et al. Neurocardiovascular instability, hypotensive episodes, and MRI lesions in neurodegenerative dementia. Ann N Y Acad Sci. 2000;903:442–5.
35. Mattace-Raso FU, Van den Meiracker AH, Bos WJ, Van der Cammen TJ, Westerhof BE, Elias-Smale S, et al. Arterial stiffness, cardiovagal baroreflex sensitivity and postural blood pressure changes in older adults: the Rotterdam study. J Hypertens. 2007;25:1421–6.
36. Van Sloten TT, Sedaghat S, Laurent S, London GM, Pannier B, Ikram MA, et al. Carotid stiffness is associated with incident stroke. a systematic review and individual participant meta-analysis J Am Coll Cardiol. 2015;66:2116–25.
37. Moretti R, Torre P, Antonello RM, et al. Risk factors for vascular dementia: hypotension as key point. Vasc Health Risk Manag. 2008;4(2):395–402.
38. Salloway S. Subcortical vascular dementia: Binswanger's and CADASIL. American Academy of Neurology (AAN). 2003. 8AC.006–2. Honolulu: 1–29.
39. Bengtsson-Lindberg M, Larsson V, Minthon L, Wattmo C, Londos E. Lack of orthostatic symptoms in dementia patients with orthostatic hypotension. Clin Auton Res. 2015;25:87–94.
40. Qiu C, Winblad B, Fratiglioni L. The age-dependent relation of blood pressure to cognitive function and dementia. Lancet Neurol. 2005;4:487–99.
41. Magnusson M, Holm H, Bachus E, Nilsson P, Leosdottir M, Melander O, et al. Orthostatic hypotension and cardiac changes after long-term follow-up. Am J Hypertens. 2016;29:847–52.
42. de Bruijn RFAG, MLP P, MJG L, Bos MJ, Hofman A, van der Lugt A, et al. Subclinical cardiac dysfunction increases the risk of stroke and dementia: the Rotterdam study. Neurology. 2015;84:833–40.
43. Jefferson AL, Beiser AS, Himali JJ, Seshadri S, O'Donnell CJ, Manning WJ, et al. Low cardiac index is associated with incident dementia and Alzheimer's disease: the Framingham heart study. Circulation. 2015;131:1333–9.
44. Andin U, Passant U, Gustafson L, Englund E. Alzheimer's disease (AD) with and without white matter pathology-clinical identification of concurrent cardiovascular disorders. Arch Gerontol Geriatr. 2007 May-Jun;44(3):277–86.
45. Räihä I, Tarvonen S, Kurki T, Rajala T, Sourander L. Relationship between vascular factors and white matter low attenuation of the brain. Acta Neurol Scand. 1993;87(4):286–9.
46. Kario K, Eguchi K, Hoshide S, Hoshide Y, Umeda Y, Mitsuhashi T, Shimada K. U-curve relationship between orthostatic blood pressure change and silent cerebrovascular disease in elderly hypertensives orthostatic hypertension as a new cardiovascular risk factor. J Am Coll Cardiol. 2002;40(1):133–41.
47. Matsubayashi K, Okumiya K, Wada T, et al. Postural dysregulation in systolic blood pressure is associated with worsened scoring on neurobehavioral function tests and leukoaraiosis in the older elderly living in a community. Stroke. 1997;28:2169–73.
48. Meng Q, Wang S, Wang Y, et al. Arterial stiffness is a potential mechanism and promising indicator of orthostatic hypotension in the general population. Vasa. 2014;43(6):423–32.
49. Suleman R, Padwal R, Hamilton P, et al. Association between central blood pressure, arterial stiffness, and mild cognitive impairment. Clin Hypertens. 2017;23:2.
50. Pase MP, Herbert A, Grima NA, et al. Arterial stiffness as a cause of cognitive decline and dementia: a systematic review and meta-analysis. Intern Med J. 2012;42:808–15.
51. van Sloten TT, Protogerou AD, Henry RN, et al. Association between arterial stiffness, cerebral small vessel disease and cognitive impairment: a systematic review and meta-analysis. Neurosci Biobehav Rev. 2015;53:121–30.
52. Idiaquez J, Rios L, Sandoval E. Postprandial hypotension in Alzheimer's disease. Clin Auton Res. 1997;7(3):119–20.
53. Idiaquez J, Benarroch EE, Rosales H, Milla P, Rios L. Autonomic and cognitive dysfunction in Parkinson's disease. Clin Auton Res. 2007;17(2):93–8.

54. Saito Y, Ishikawa J, Harada K. Postprandial and orthostatic hypotension treated by Sitagliptin in a patient with dementia with Lewy bodies. The American Journal of Case Reports. 2016;17:887–93. https://doi.org/10.12659/AJCR.900620.
55. Kenny RA, Shaw FE, O' Brien JT, Scheltens PH, Kalaria R, Ballard C. Carotid sinus syndrome is common in dementia with Lewy bodies and correlates with deep white matter lesions. J Neurol Neurosurg Psychiatry. 2004;75(7):966–71.
56. Miller VM, Kenny RA, Slade JY, Oakley AF, Kalaria RN. Medullary autonomic pathology in carotid sinus hypersensitivity. Neuropathol Appl Neurobiol. 2008;34(4):403–11.
57. Kenny RA, Kalaria R, Ballard C. Neurocardiovascular instability in cognitive impairment and dementia. Ann N Y Acad Sci. 2002 Nov;977:183–95.
58. Ballard C, O'Brien J, Barber B, Scheltens P, Shaw F, McKeith I, Kenny RA. Neurocardiovascular instability, hypotensive episodes, and MRI lesions in neurodegenerative dementia. Ann N Y Acad Sci. 2000;903:442–5.
59. Schoon Y, Lagro J, Verhoeven Y, Rikkert MO, Claassen J. Hypotensive syndromes are not associated with cognitive impairment in geriatric patients. Am J Alzheimers Dis Other Dement. 2013;28(1):47–53.
60. Frewen J, King-kallimanis B, Boyle G, Kenny RA. Recent syncope and unexplained falls are associated with poor cognitive performance. Age Ageing. 2015;44(2):282–6.
61. Romero SA, Minson CT, Halliwal JR. The cardiovascular system after exercise. J Appl Physiol. 1985;122(4):925–32.
62. Erickson KI, Kramer AF. Aerobic exercise effects on cognitive and neural plasticity in older adults. Br J Sports Med. 2009;43(1):22–4.
63. Makizako H, Liu-Ambrose T, Shimada H, et al. Moderate-intensity physical activity, hippocampal volume, and memory in older adults with mild cognitive impairment. J Gerontol A Biol Sci Med Sci. 2014;70(4):480–6.
64. Colcombe SJ, Kramer AF, Erickson KI, et al. Cardiovascular fitness, cortical plasticity, and aging. Proc Natl Acad Sci U S A. 2004;101(9):3316–21.
65. Guo H, Tabara Y, Igase M, et al. Abnormal nocturnal blood pressure profile is associated with mild cognitive impairment in the elderly: the J- Shipp study. Hypertens Res. 2010;33:32–6.
66. Borson S, Scanlan JM, Chen P, et al. The mini-cog as a screen for dementia: validation in a population-base sample. J Am Geriatr Soc. 2003;51:1451–4.
67. Molloy DW, Standish TIM. A guide to the standardized mini-mental state examination. Int Psychogeriatr. 1997;9(1):87–94.
68. Nasreddine ZS, Phillips NA, Bédirian V, et al. The Montreal cognitive assessment, MoCA: a brief screening tool for mild cognitive impairment. J Am Geriatr Soc. 2005;53(4):695–9.
69. Tariq SH, Tumosa N, Chibnall JT, et al. Comparison of the Saint Louis university mental status examination and the mini-mental state examination for detecting dementia and mild neurocognitive disorder – a pilot study. Am J Geriatr Psychiatry. 2006;14:900–10.
70. Brodaty H, Pond D, Kemp NM, et al. The GPCOG: a new screening test for dementia designed for general practice. J Am Geriatr Soc. 2002;50:530–4.
71. Dubois B, Slachevsky A, Litvan I, et al. The FAB. A frontal assessment battery at bedside. Neurology. 2000;55:1621–6.
72. Bassuk SS, Murphy JM. Characteristics of the modified mini-mental state exam among elderly persons. J Clin Epidemiol. 2003;56:622–8.
73. Teng EL, Hasegawa K, Homma A, et al. The cognitive abilities screening instrument (CASI): a practical test for cross-cultural epidemiological studies of dementia. Int Psychogeriatr. 1994;6(1):45–58.
74. Ames H, Hendrickse WA, Bakshi RS, et al. Utility of the neurobehavioral cognitive status examination (Cognistat) with geriatric mental health outpatients. Clin Gerontol. 2009;32(2):198–210.
75. Stokholm J, Vogel A, Gade A. The executive interview as a screening test for executive dysfunction in patients with mild dementia. J Am Geriatr Soc. 2005;53(9):1577–81.
76. Petersen RC. Clinical practice. Mild cognitive impairment. N Engl J Med. 2011;364: 2227–34.

77. Portet F, Ousset PJ, Visser PJ, et al. Mild cognitive impairment (MCI) in medical practice: a critical review of the concept and new diagnostic procedure. Report of the MCI working Group of the European Consortium on Alzheimer's disease. J Neurol Neurosurg Psychiatry. 2006;77:714–8.
78. American Psychiatric Association. Diagnostic and statistical manual of mental disorders, fourth edition (DSM-IV). Washington, DC, USA: American Psychiatric Association; 2004.
79. McKhann G, Drachman D, Folstein M, et al. Clinical diagnosis of Alzheimer's disease: report of the NINCDS-ADRDA work group under the auspices of Department of Health and Human Services Task Force on Alzheimer's disease. Neurology. 1984;34(7):939–44.
80. Roman GC, Tatemichi TK, Erkinjuntti T, et al. Vascular dementia: diagnostic criteria for research studies: report of the NINDS-AIREN international workshop. Neurology. 1993;43:250–60.
81. Hughes CP, Berg L, Danziger WL, et al. A new clinical scale for the staging of dementia. Br J Psychiatry. 1982 Jun;140:566–72.

Index

© Springer Nature Switzerland AG 2020
K. Alagiakrishnan, M. Banach (eds.), *Hypotensive Syndromes in Geriatric
Patients*, https://doi.org/10.1007/978-3-030-30332-7